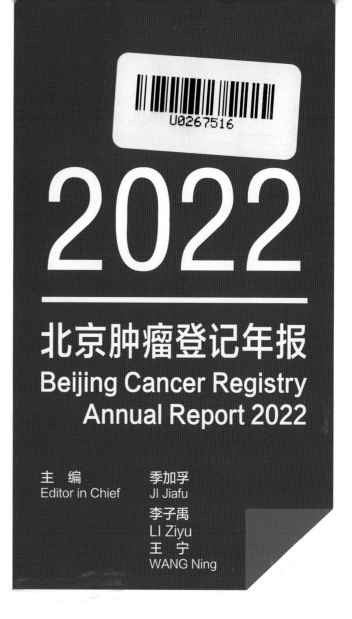

2022

北京肿瘤登记年报
Beijing Cancer Registry
Annual Report 2022

主 编	季加孚
Editor in Chief	JI Jiafu
	李子禹
	LI Ziyu
	王 宁
	WANG Ning

北京大学医学出版社

2022 BEIJING ZHONGLIU DENGJI NIANBAO

图书在版编目（CIP）数据

2022 北京肿瘤登记年报 / 季加孚，李子禹，王宁主编 . —北京：北京大学医学出版社，2023.4
ISBN 978-7-5659-2814-7

Ⅰ. ① 2… Ⅱ. ①季… ②李… ③王… Ⅲ. ①肿瘤－卫生统计－北京－2022－年报 Ⅳ. ① R73-54

中国国家版本馆 CIP 数据核字（2023）第 006090 号

审图号：京 S（2023）009 号

2022 北京肿瘤登记年报

主 编：季加孚 李子禹 王 宁
出版发行：北京大学医学出版社
地 址：（100191）北京市海淀区学院路 38 号 北京大学医学部院内
电 话：发行部 010-82802230；图书邮购 010-82802495
网 址：http://www.pumpress.com.cn
E - mail：booksale@bjmu.edu.cn
印 刷：北京信彩瑞禾印刷厂
经 销：新华书店
责任编辑：董采萱 责任校对：靳新强 责任印制：李 啸
开 本：889 mm×1194 mm 1/16 印张：15.5 字数：340 千字
版 次：2023 年 4 月第 1 版 2023 年 4 月第 1 次印刷
书 号：ISBN 978-7-5659-2814-7
定 价：185.00 元

前　言

　　恶性肿瘤是严重威胁居民生命和健康的一大类疾病，多年来一直是北京市居民的主要死亡原因，且发病呈现逐年上升趋势。肿瘤登记是定期收集某地人群恶性肿瘤发病、死亡和生存数据的系统性工作，是制定肿瘤防治政策、评价防控效果及开展相关研究的基础性疾病监测工作。北京市卫生健康委员会发布的关于贯彻落实《健康中国行动——癌症防治实施方案（2019—2022年）》有关工作的通知中明确指出，要"强化肿瘤登记报告工作，提高报告效率及质量"。

　　肿瘤登记工作的标志性成果之一就是每年及时向政府和社会发布北京市肿瘤登记监测数据。近年来，北京市肿瘤登记监测数据不仅被国际癌症研究署和国际肿瘤登记协会《五大洲癌症发病率》收录出版，标志着北京市肿瘤登记数据达到国际水平，而且自2010年起由北京市政府通过《北京市卫生与人群健康状况报告》向社会公布，体现了政府对人民健康和肿瘤防治工作的重视。本年报汇总了2019年北京市恶性肿瘤监测数据，包含23种恶性肿瘤及所有恶性肿瘤合计的发病和死亡数据，同时分地区、年龄和性别比较了恶性肿瘤的分布差异。

　　《2022北京肿瘤登记年报》的顺利完成，得到了国家癌症中心/全国肿瘤登记中心、北京市卫生健康委员会疾病预防控制处、北京市疾病预防控制中心、北京市卫生健康大数据与政策研究中心和北京大学肿瘤医院的大力支持，凝结着全市近200家医疗机构工作人员的辛苦付出和30余位编写、校审人员的辛勤劳动。它的出版发行得益于所有工作人员的支持和付出，在此表示衷心的感谢！

北京市肿瘤防治研究办公室　主任

中国抗癌协会　副理事长

2022年10月

Foreword

Cancer is a group of numerous distinct disease that intimidates mankind's life and health seriously and has been the leading cause of deaths in Beijing for many years. The incidence of cancer in Beijing also increased gradually in recent years.

Cancer registration is a systematic work that collects cancer incidence, mortality and survival data for a specific population at regular intervals. Cancer registration is a basic surveillance work which plays an important role for formulating cancer prevention policies, evaluating the impact of cancer prevention and control, and supplying basic evidence for related research. In the notice on implementing *Healthy China Action: Action Plan for Cancer Prevention and Control (2019-2022)* issued by Beijing Municipal Health Commission emphasized on strengthening cancer registration and improving efficacy and quality of data submission.

One prominent achievement of cancer registration in Beijing is to release Beijing cancer surveillance data to public. In recent years, the cancer surveillance data in Beijing has been accepted by *Cancer Incidence in Five Continents* published by the International Agency for Research on Cancer (IARC) and International Association of Cancer Registries (IACR), which marked the quality of data in Beijing reached the international level. And the cancer surveillance data have been issued to public through the *Health and Population Health Report of Beijing* by the Municipal Government of Beijing since 2010, which indicates that the government attaches great importance to people's health and cancer prevention and control. In this report, cancer incidence and mortality data in Beijing of 2019 were reported, including summarized data of the incidence and mortality for cancer combined and 23 cancer sites. Area-, age- and sex- specific characteristics were also calculated.

National Cancer Center & National Central Cancer Registry, Division of Disease Prevention and Control of the Beijing Municipal Health Commission, Beijing Center for Disease Prevention and Control, Beijing Municipal Health Big Data and Policy Research Center and Peking University Cancer Hospital provided sustainable support in publication of the *Beijing Cancer Registry Annual Report 2022*. And it also embodies the hard work of staffs from nearly 200 medical institutions and more than 30 authors and editors.

I acknowledge the support and dedication of all the staffs who contributed to this publication.

Director of Beijing Office for Cancer Prevention and Control

Deputy President of China Anti-cancer Association

October, 2022

目录

Contents

1 概述
Introduction

1.1 北京市肿瘤登记处概况

北京市肿瘤登记处始建于 1977 年，2010 年归入北京市肿瘤防治研究办公室，隶属于北京市卫生健康委员会疾病预防控制处管理，挂靠在北京大学肿瘤医院和北京市肿瘤防治研究所。目前，登记处有 7 名专职工作人员，其中博士 4 人，硕士 3 人。

北京市面积为 16 411 平方公里，位于北纬 39°56′，东经 116°20′，属于暖温带半湿润半干旱季风气候，年平均年降水量为 450~750 mm，年平均相对湿度为 50%。北京市肿瘤登记处收集的发病和死亡数据覆盖全市 16 个区的 1 368 万人口，其中 95.2% 是汉族，少数民族只占 4.8%。

北京是中华人民共和国的首都，也是政治、经济和文化中心，医疗技术水平国内领先，医疗设备完善。2019 年北京市卫生健康委员会管辖的二级及以上医疗机构中，177 家报告肿瘤病例（其中肿瘤专科医院 9 家），其余医院不收治肿瘤患者。

北京市肿瘤登记处通过"北京市卫生综合统计信息平台"收集各医院上报的肿瘤发病和死亡数据。北京市肿瘤死亡信息由北京市疾病预防控制中心的生命统计部门提供，人口资料由北京市公安局提供。

1.1 Brief introduction of Beijing Cancer Registry（BCR）

BCR was founded in 1977 and was merged into the Beijing Office for Cancer Prevention and Control, which was affiliated to the Division of Disease Prevention and Control of the Beijing Municipal Health Commission in 2010. It also belongs to Peking University Cancer Hospital and the Beijing Institute for Cancer Research. At present, there are seven full-time employees working with the registry（4 have Ph.D. degree and 3 have Master degree）.

Beijing is located at the latitude of 39° 56′ N, and the longitude of 116° 20′ E, covering 16,411 square kilometers. It belongs to the warm temperate zone, semi-humid and semi-arid monsoon climate. The average annual precipitation is about 450-750 mm, with the relative humidity 50%. The BCR covers the 16 administrative districts of Beijing, with about 13.68 million inhabitants, 95.2% of whom are Han Chinese and 4.8% from ethnic minority groups.

Beijing, the capital and the political, economic and cultural center of China, boasts the top-notch healthcare facilities equipped with cutting-edge technologies of the country. Among the secondary and tertiary hospitals under the supervision of the Beijing Municipal Health Commission, 177 hospitals have reported cancer case information to the BCR in 2019, including 9 cancer hospitals. The other hospitals that do not treat and report cancer patients were not included into the surveillance.

The BCR collects cancer incidence and mortality data from the "Beijing Health-care Information Statistical Platform" provided by the Beijing Municipal Health Commission. The mortality data are derived from the vital statistics department of the Beijing Center for Disease Prevention and Control, and the population data are provided by the Beijing Municipal Public Security Bureau.

1.2 北京市肿瘤登记体系建设及发展历史

肿瘤登记是定期收集某地人群癌症数据的系统性工作，收集的信息包括癌症患者个人信息、诊断信息、治疗信息、随访信息和当地人口资料。肿瘤登记是制定癌症防控政策、评价癌症防控效果及开展相关研究的基础性疾病监测工作。

北京市自 1977 年根据《关于建立北京市恶性肿瘤登记报告制度及进行死亡回顾调查的通知》[（76）京卫科学第 191 号] 文件要求，开展以人群为基础的肿瘤登记工作以来，最初在城区采用（东城、西城、崇文、宣武、朝阳、海淀、丰台、石景山）医院手工填写报告卡的方式报告首诊病例。20 世纪 90 年代逐步覆盖全市 16 区，并以北京市疾病预防控制中心生命统计部门提供的死亡资料作为发病漏报和死亡结局的补充。2004 年根据《关于加强和落实北京市肿瘤登记报告工作的通知》（京卫办字［2004］39 号文件），开始通过"北京市卫生综合统计信息平台"的肿瘤登记模块，每月采集全市二级及以上医疗机构的出院病案首页信息，收集恶性肿瘤患者信息，实现了全市网络直报，减少了漏报率，提高了时效性。

2009 年北京市开展覆盖全市的病案核查工作，逐步提高形态学确诊（morphological verification, MV）比例，降低部位不明（other and unspecified sites, O&U）比例和仅有死亡医学证明书（death certificate only, DCO）的比例。2010 年，为了准确评估北京市户籍居民癌症患者的生存状况，北京市针对肿瘤现患患者开展主动随访工作，并延续至今。

1.2 Development history of the cancer registration system in Beijing

Cancer registration is a systematic work that collects cancer data for a specific population at regular intervals. The information being collected includes the demographic, diagnosis, treatment, follow-up and the population data. Cancer registration is a basic surveillance work which plays an important role for formulating cancer prevention policies, evaluating the impact of cancer prevention and control, and supplying basic evidence for related research.

The BCR was founded according to the administrative document of *Establishing Beijing Cancer Registration and Conducting Retrospective Investigation on Death*. The BCR has been collecting population-based cancer information using the manually filled report cards since 1977. The surveillance covered 8 urban districts: Dongcheng, Xicheng, Chongwen, Xuanwu, Chaoyang, Haidian, Fengtai and Shijingshan. In the 1990s, the coverage of the surveillance was gradually expanded, covering all the 16 districts of the city, and supplementary information—the death certificate information from the vital statistics department of the Beijing Centers for Disease Prevention and Control, was used as a source for missed reporting of cases and the mortality data. According to the administrative document of *Strengthening Data Reporting and Application of Beijing Cancer Registration*, since 2004, we have been using the cancer registration system, a module of the "Beijing Health-care Information Statistical Platform", to collect the patient information monthly from the profile information of the medical records of patients discharged from secondary or tertiary hospitals in Beijing. This made direct online reporting possible, reducing the rate of underreporting and improving the timeliness of data reporting.

In 2009, the BCR re-abstracted the medical record of all related facilities in Beijing to raise the proportion of morphological verified cases (MV%), to reduce the proportion of "other and unspecified cases" (O&U%) and the proportion of cancer cases recognized by death certificate only (DCO%). In order to accurately evaluate the survival of cancer patients with Beijing households, the BCR has been following up cancer patients who are still alive in Beijing since 2010.

1.3 年报统计数据

1.3.1 年报数据收集范围

本年报数据收集截止时间为 2022 年 6 月 30 日，数据上报时间范围为 2019 年 1 月 1 日至 2019 年 12 月 31 日，上报医院共计 177 家北京市二级及以上医疗机构。ICD-10（国际疾病分类第 10 版，International Classification of Diseases 10th Revision）编码收集范围为 C00-97、D00-09、D32-33、D42-43、D45-47，经过核查病历剔除良性肿瘤和原位癌，年报 ICD-10 编码统计范围为 C00-97 和 D45-47。人口数据采用 2019 年年中人口数据，覆盖北京市 16 区户籍人口 13 866 241 人（男性 6 894 578 人，女性 6 971 663 人），其中城区 6 个（东城、西城、朝阳、海淀、丰台、石景山，2010 年崇文和宣武分别并入东城和西城），覆盖人口 8 543 242 人，占 61.61%；郊区 10 个（门头沟、房山、通州、顺义、昌平、大兴、怀柔、平谷、密云、延庆），覆盖人口 5 322 999 人，占 38.39%。

1.3.2 年报主要统计内容

本年报汇总了北京市 16 区户籍人口的癌症发病、死亡数据及人口数据。详细描述了北京市肿瘤登记处数据的质量控制指标结果，如 MV%、M/I、DCO%、O&U% 等。详细报道了合计癌症和 23 种癌症的发病与死亡数据，指标包括：发病率，死亡率，中国人口标化率（2000 年中国人口构成），世界人口标化率（Segi 世界标准人口构成），累积率，分城郊、年龄组、性别的发病率及死亡率等。部分癌种按亚部位和组织学分型进行了细节描述。

1.3 Data specification in this annual report

1.3.1 Data collection scope

Medical records of newly diagnosed cancer patients and deaths from all the 177 hospitals between Jan.1, 2019 and Dec. 31, 2019 were reported to the BCR by Jun. 30, 2022. According to the International Classification of Diseases 10th Revision（ICD-10）, the cases with the codes of C00-97, D32-33, D42-43, and D45-47 were included into the BCR surveillance system, but only the cases with the codes of C00-97 and D45-47 were included into analysis in this annual report after excluding the benign tumors recognized through medical record verification. The Beijing population in the middle of 2019 was used for incidence and mortality calculation in this annual report. At that time, there were 13,866,241 permanent residents in Beijing（6,894,578 males, 6,971,663 females, respectively）, with 8,543,242 residents（61.61%）from the 6 urban districts（Dongcheng, Xicheng, Chaoyang, Haidian, Fengtai, and Shijingshan; Chongwen and Xuanwu were merged into Dongcheng and Xicheng, respectively, in 2010）and 5,322,999 residents（38.39%）from the 10 peri-urban districts（Mentougou, Fangshan, Tongzhou, Shunyi, Changping,Daxing, Huairou, Pinggu, Miyun, and Yanqing）.

1.3.2 Contents of this annual report

The present annual report summarizes the data of the cancer incidence and mortality of all the permanent residents and the population data of the 16 districts in Beijing. We report the quality control indicators in details, including the proportion of morphological verified cases（MV%）, the mortality to incidence ratio（M/I）, the proportion of cases recognized by death certificate only（DCO%）, and the proportion of "other and unspecified cases"（O&U%）. We report data of new cases and deaths of all cancers and by 23 main sites, including crude incidence, mortality, age-standardized rates（ASRs）of the Chinese population in 2000, ASRs of Segi's world standardized population, cumulative rates, age-specific rates, and sex-specific rates. Moreover, the characteristics of subsites and morphological sub-types for specific cancers were also calculated and described.

（撰稿 王宁，校稿 杨雷）

2 资料来源、收集方法与质量控制
Data Source, Collection Methods and Quality Control

2.1 北京市以人群为基础的肿瘤登记资料收集方法

北京市肿瘤登记资料的收集采用被动和主动两种方法。被动收集是指各医院定期报送肿瘤病例资料，或肿瘤登记处从死因监测部门获取肿瘤患者死亡信息。主动收集是指到医院查阅肿瘤病例的诊疗病史，摘录肿瘤病历信息，或主动随访以获取肿瘤患者的生存信息。

2.1.1 北京市肿瘤登记资料的主要来源

北京市二级及以上医疗机构（表 2.1.1）每月将住院肿瘤患者的发病和死亡信息通过"北京市卫生综合统计信息平台"报送至北京市肿瘤登记处。

死亡病例的主要来源为北京市疾病预防控制中心生命统计部门提供的肿瘤患者死亡数据库。此数据库同时作为补充肿瘤登记发病资料漏报的重要渠道。

对于肿瘤登记数据库中仍存活病例（现患病例），将通过社区主动随访的形式进一步补充可能的死亡结局。

人口资料来源于北京市公安局的人口统计资料，标准人口结构来源于人口普查资料和 Segi 世界标准人口结构。

2.1 Methods of the data collection from population-based cancer registry of Beijing

We adopted passive and active data collection methods. Passive collection was defined as reporting of the information of the diagnosed cancer patients by the hospitals to the registry at regular intervals or linking the data file of the vital statistics derived from the responsible department. Active collection happened when the registry retrieved the cancer data proactively from medical record departments of the hospitals, or followed up the cancer patients in the communities for the survival status.

2.1.1 Data sources of the Beijing Cancer Registry

Cancer incidence and mortality data from the health institutions (secondary and above, Table 2.1.1) were submitted to the BCR monthly using the Beijing Health-care Information Statistical Platform.

The death certificate data were derived from the cancer patient mortality database of the vital statistics department of the Beijing Center for Disease Prevention and Control. The database was also used as an important supplementary source to improve the completeness of the data.

The patients that were still recorded as alive in the database were followed-up proactively at the community level.

The population data were provided by the Beijing Municipal Public Security Bureau. The standard age structure of the population was based on the China population census data and Segi's world standardized population structure.

表 2.1.1 2019 年北京市报告肿瘤登记资料的医疗机构
Table 2.1.1 The medical institutions which submitted cancer case data in Beijing, 2019

辖区 District	医疗机构数 No. of medical institutions	医疗机构名称 Name of medical institutions
北京市 Beijing	1	北京市疾病预防控制中心 Beijing Center for Disease Prevention and Control
东城区 Dongcheng	15	中国医学科学院北京协和医院 Peking Union Medical College Hospital
		北京医院 Beijing Hospital
		首都医科大学附属北京同仁医院 Beijing Tongren Hospital, Capital Medical University
		首都医科大学附属北京妇产医院 Beijing Obstetrics and Gynecology Hospital, Capital Medical University
		首都医科大学附属北京中医医院 Beijing Hospital of Traditional Chinese Medicine, Capital Medical University
		北京市普仁医院 Beijing Puren Hospital
		北京中医药大学东直门医院 Dongzhimen Hospital, Beijing University of Chinese Medicine
		北京市隆福医院（北京市东城区老年病医院） Beijing Longfu Hospital （Beijing Dongcheng Geriatric Hospital）
		北京市第六医院 Beijing No.6 Hospital
		北京市和平里医院 Beijing Hepingli Hospital
		首都医科大学附属北京口腔医院 Beijing Stomatological Hospital, Capital Medical University
		北京市东城区第一人民医院 Beijing Dongcheng District First People's Hospital
		北京市鼓楼中医医院 Beijing Gulou Traditional Chinese Medicine Hospital
		北京同仁堂中医医院 Beijing Tongrentang Hospital of Traditional Chinese Medicine
		北京市东城区妇幼保健计划生育服务中心 Beijing Dongcheng Maternal and Child Health and Family Planning Service Center
西城区 Xicheng	21	北京大学人民医院 Peking University People's Hospital
		北京大学第一医院 Peking University First Hospital

续表

辖区 District	医疗机构数 No. of medical institutions	医疗机构名称 Name of medical institutions
西城区 Xicheng	21	首都医科大学附属北京友谊医院 Beijing Friendship Hospital, Capital Medical University
		首都医科大学附属北京儿童医院 Beijing Children's Hospital, Capital Medical University
		首都医科大学宣武医院 Xuanwu Hospital, Capital Medical University
		北京积水潭医院 Beijing Jishuitan Hospital
		中国中医科学院广安门医院 Guang'anmen Hospital, China Academy of Chinese Medical Sciences
		首都医科大学附属复兴医院 Fuxing Hospital, Capital Medical University
		北京市健宫医院 Beijing Jiangong Hospital
		北京市肛肠医院 Beijing Rectum Hospital
		北京市回民医院 Beijing Huimin Hospital
		北京市西城区展览路医院 Zhanlanlu Hospital of Xicheng District, Beijing
		北京中医药大学附属护国寺中医医院 Huguosi Hospital of Traditional Chinese Medicine of Beijing University of Chinese Medicine
		北京市宣武中医医院 Beijing Xuanwu Traditional Chinese Medical Hospital
		北京市西城区广外医院 Guangwai Hospital of Xicheng District, Beijing
		北京市监狱管理局中心医院 Beijing Prison Administration Central Hospital
		北京市第二医院 The Second Hospital of Beijing
		北京市西城区平安医院 Ping'an Hospital of Xicheng District, Beijing
		中国医学科学院阜外医院 Fuwai Hospital, Chinese Academy of Medical Sciences
		北京新世纪儿童医院 New Century International Children's Hospital

续表

辖区 District	医疗机构数 No. of medical institutions	医疗机构名称 Name of medical institutions
西城区 Xicheng	21	北京市丰盛中医骨伤专科医院 Beijing Fengsheng Special Hospital of Traditional Medical Traumatology and Orthopaedics
朝阳区 Chaoyang	31	中国医学科学院肿瘤医院 Cancer Hospital, Chinese Academy of Medical Sciences
		中日友好医院 China-Japan Friendship Hospital
		首都医科大学附属北京朝阳医院 Beijing Chao-Yang Hospital, Capital Medical University
		首都医科大学附属北京地坛医院 Beijing Ditan Hospital, Capital Medical University
		北京朝阳中西医结合急诊抢救中心 Beijing Chaoyang Integrative Medicine Emergency Medical Center
		首都儿科研究所附属儿童医院 Children's Hospital, Capital Institute of Pediatrics
		首都医科大学附属北京安贞医院 Beijing Anzhen Hospital, Capital Medical University
		民航总医院 Civil Aviation General Hospital
		北京华信医院（清华大学第一附属医院） Beijing Huaxin Hospital（The First Hospital of Tsinghua University）
		应急管理部应急总医院 Emergency General Hospital
		航空总医院 Aviation General Hospital
		北京市垂杨柳医院 Beijing Chui Yang Liu Hospital
		中国中医科学院望京医院 Wangjing Hospital of China Academy of Chinese Medical Sciences
		北京中医药大学第三附属医院 Beijing University of Chinese Medicine Third Affiliated Hospital
		北京市第一中西医结合医院 Beijing First Integrated Traditional Chinese and Western Medicine Hospital
		北京市朝阳区中医医院 Beijing Chaoyang Hospital of Traditional Chinese Medicine
		北京和睦家医院 Beijing United Family Hospital

续表

辖区 District	医疗机构数 No. of medical institutions	医疗机构名称 Name of medical institutions
朝阳区 Chaoyang	31	北京市朝阳区妇幼保健院 Beijing Chaoyang Maternal and Child Health Care Hospital
		北京市朝阳区双桥医院 Shuangqiao Hospital of Chaoyang District, Beijing
		北京伟达中医肿瘤医院 Beijing Weida Tumor Hospital of Traditional Chinese Medicine
		北京市红十字会急诊抢救中心 Beijing Red Cross Society Emergency Rescue Center
		首都机场集团紧急医学救援中心 Emergency Medical Rescue Centre of the Capital Airport Group
		北京五洲妇儿医院 GlobalCare Women and Children's Hospital
		北京四惠中医医院 Beijing Sihui Hospital of Traditional Chinese Medicine
		北京百子湾和美妇儿医院 HarMoniCare Beijing Women and Children's Hospital（Baiziwan）
		北京和美妇儿医院 HarMoniCare Beijing Women and Children's Hospital
		中国藏学研究中心北京藏医院 Beijng Tibetan Medicine Hospital, China Tibetology Research Center
		北京和平里中西医结合医院 Beijing Hepingli Hospital of Integrated Traditional and Western Medicine
		北京市朝阳区桓兴肿瘤医院 Cancer Hospital of Huanxing ChaoYang District, Beijing
		北京市朝阳区三环肿瘤医院 Sanhuan Cancer Hospital of Chaoyang District, Beijing
		北京精诚博爱医院 Beijing Jingcheng Bo'ai Hospital
丰台区 Fengtai	25	首都医科大学附属北京天坛医院 Beijing Tiantan Hospital, Capital Medical University
		首都医科大学附属北京佑安医院 Beijing You'an Hospital, Capital Medical University
		北京中医药大学东方医院 Dongfang Hospital, Beijing University of Chinese Medicine
		北京航天总医院 Beijing Aerospace General Hospital
		国家电网公司北京电力医院 Beijing Electric Power Hospital

续表

辖区 District	医疗机构数 No. of medical institutions	医疗机构名称 Name of medical institutions
丰台区 Fengtai	25	北京瑶医医院 Beijing Yao Medicine Hospital
		北京丰台右安门医院 Beijing Fengtai You'anmen Hospital
		北京高博博仁医院 Beijing GoBroad Boren Hospital
		中国航天科工集团七三一医院 AMHT Group Aerospace 731 Hospital
		北京欧亚肿瘤医院 Beijing Ouya Cancer Hospital
		北京丰台医院 Beijing Fengtai Hospital
		北京京西肿瘤医院 Western Beijing Cancer Hospital
		北京博爱医院 Beijing Bo'ai Hospital
		北京市丰台中西医结合医院 Beijing Fengtai Hospital of Integrated Traditional and Western Medicine
		北京市丰台区中医医院 Beijing Fengtai Hospital of Traditional Chinese Medicine
		北京长峰医院 Beijing Changfeng Hospital
		北京市丰台区老年人协会莲花池康复医院 Beijing Lianhuachi Rehabilitation Hospital
		北京市丰台区妇幼保健计划生育服务中心 Beijing Fengtai Maternal and Child Health and Family Planning Service Center
		北京华坛中西医结合医院 Beijing Huatan Integrative Medicine Hospital
		北京汇安中西医结合医院 Beijing Hui'an Hospital of Integrated Traditional and Western Hospital
		北京市红十字会和平骨科医院 Beijing Red Cross Society Heping Orthopedic Hospital
		北京市木材厂职工医院 Beijing Timber Factory Worker's Hospital
		北京六一八厂医院 Beijing 618 Factory Hospital

续表

辖区 District	医疗机构数 No. of medical institutions	医疗机构名称 Name of medical institutions
丰台区 Fengtai	25	北京首大眼耳鼻喉医院 Shouda Eye and E.N.T Hospital of Beijing
		北京市丰台康复医院（铁营医院） Fengtai Rehabilitation Hospotal of Beijing Municipality（Tieying Hospital）
石景山区 Shijingshan	7	北京大学首钢医院 Peking University Shougang Hospital
		北京市石景山医院 Beijing Shijingshan Hospital
		清华大学玉泉医院（清华大学中西医结合医院） Yuquan Hospital Affiliated to Tsinghua University（Integrated Traditional Chinese and Western Medicine Hospital of Tsinghua University）
		首都医科大学附属北京康复医院 Beijing Rehabilitation Hospital, Capital Medical University
		中国中医科学院眼科医院 Eye Hospital, China Academy of Chinese Medical Sciences
		北京联科中医肾病医院 Beijing United-Tech Nephrology Specialist Hospital
		中国医学科学院整形外科医院 Plastic Surgery Hospital of Chinese Academy of Medical Sciences
海淀区 Haidian	19	北京肿瘤医院 Beijing Cancer Hospital
		北京大学第三医院 Peking University Third Hospital
		首都医科大学附属北京世纪坛医院 Beijing Shijitan Hospital, Capital Medical University
		航天中心医院 Aerospace Center Hospital
		首都医科大学三博脑科医院 Sanbo Brain Hospital, Capital Medical University
		中国中医科学院西苑医院 Xiyuan Hospital, China Academy of Chinese Medical Sciences
		北京市海淀医院 Beijing Haidian Hospital
		北京大学口腔医院 Peking University Hospital of Stomatology
		北京老年医院 Beijing Geriatric Hospital

辖区 District	医疗机构数 No. of medical institutions	医疗机构名称 Name of medical institutions
海淀区 Haidian	19	北京市中关村医院（中国科学院中关村医院） Beijing Zhongguancun Hospital （Zhongguancun Hospital of Chinese Academy of Sciences）
		北京中西医结合医院 Beijing Hospital of Integrated Traditional Chinese and Western Medicine
		北京市海淀区妇幼保健院 Beijing Haidian Maternal and Child Health Care Hospital
		北京裕和中西医结合康复医院 Beijing Yuho Rehabilitation Hospital
		北京水利医院 Beijing Water Conservancy Hospital
		北京四季青医院 Beijing Sijiqing Hospital
		北京大学医院 Peking University Hospital
		清华大学医院 Tsinghua University Hospital
		北京市上地医院 Beijing Shangdi Hospital
		北京德尔康尼骨科医院 Beijing Diakonie Orthopaedic Hospital
门头沟区 Mentougou	4	北京京煤集团总医院 Beijing Jingmei Group General Hospital
		北京市门头沟区医院 Beijing Mentougou District Hospital
		北京市门头沟区妇幼保健计划生育服务中心 Beijing Mentougou Maternal and Child Health and Family Planning Service Center
		北京市门头沟区中医医院 Beijing Mentougou Hospital of Traditional Chinese Medicine
房山区 Fangshan	7	北京燕化医院 Beijing Yanhua Hospital
		北京市房山区良乡医院 Liangxiang Hospital, Fangshan District, Beijing
		北京市房山区第一医院 The Frist Hospital of Fangshan District, Beijing
		北京核工业医院 Beijing Nuclear Industry Hospital

辖区 District	医疗机构数 No. of medical institutions	医疗机构名称 Name of medical institutions
房山区 Fangshan	7	北京市房山区中医医院（北京中医药大学房山医院） Beijing Fangshan Hospital of Traditional Chinese Medicine（Fangshan Hospital，Beijing University of Chinese Medicine）
		北京市房山区妇幼保健院 Beijing Fangshan Maternal and Child Health Care Hospital
		北京北亚骨科医院 Beijing Beiya Orthopedics Hospital
通州区 Tongzhou	6	首都医科大学附属北京胸科医院 Beijing Chest Hospital, Capital Medical University
		首都医科大学附属北京潞河医院 Beijing Luhe Hospital, Capital Medical University
		北京市通州区中医医院 Beijing Tongzhou Hospital of Traditional Chinese Medicine
		北京市通州区妇幼保健院 Beijing Tongzhou Maternal and Child Health Care Hospital
		北京市通州区中西医结合医院 Beijing Tongzhou Hospital of Integrated Traditional Chinese and Western Medicine
		首都医科大学附属北京友谊医院（通州院区） Beijing Friendship Hospital, Capital Medical University（Tongzhou）
顺义区 Shunyi	5	北京市顺义区医院 Beijing Shunyi Hospital
		北京市顺义区妇幼保健院（北京儿童医院顺义妇儿医院） Beijing Shunyi Maternal and Child Health Care Hospital（Shunyi Women's & Children's Hospital of Beijing Children's Hospital）
		北京市顺义区中医医院（北京中医医院顺义医院） Beijing Shunyi Hospital of Traditional Chinese Medicine（Shunyi Hospital of Beijing Chinese Medicine Hospital）
		北京市顺义区空港医院 Beijing Shunyi Airport Hospital
		首都医科大学附属北京地坛医院（顺义院区） Beijing Ditan Hospital, Capital Medical University（Shunyi）
昌平区 Changping	14	北京大学国际医院 Peking University International Hospital
		北京清华长庚医院 Beijing Tsinghua Changgung Hospital
		北京京都儿童医院 Beijing Jingdu Children's Hospital

辖区 District	医疗机构数 No. of medical institutions	医疗机构名称 Name of medical institutions
昌平区 Changping	14	北京市昌平区医院 Beijing Changping Hospital
		北京王府中西医结合医院 Beijing Royal Integrative Medicine Hospital
		北京市昌平区中医医院 Beijing Changping Hospital of Traditional Chinese Medicine
		北京市昌平区中西医结合医院 Beijing Changping Hospital of Integrated Chinese and Western Medicine
		北京大卫中医医院 Beijing David Chinese Medicine Hospital
		北京市昌平区沙河医院 Shahe Hospital, Changping District, Beijing
		北京市昌平区妇幼保健院 Beijing Changping Maternal and Child Health Care Hospital
		北京市昌平区南口医院 Nankou Hospital, Changping District, Beijing
		北京小汤山医院 Beijing Xiaotangshan Hospital
		北京北大医疗康复医院 PKUCare Rehabilitation Hospital
		北京回龙观医院 Beijing Huilongguan Hospital
大兴区 Daxing	9	北京南郊肿瘤医院 Beijing Nanjiao Cancer Hospital
		北京市大兴区人民医院 Renmin Hospital of Daxing District, Beijing
		北京市仁和医院 Beijing Renhe Hospital
		中国中医科学院广安门医院南区 Guang'anmen Hospital, China Academy of Chinese Medical Sciences（South）
		北京市大兴区中西医结合医院 Beijing Daxing District Hospital of Integrated Chinese and Western Medicine
		北京陆道培医院 Beijing Lu Daopei Hospital
		北京市大兴区妇幼保健院 Beijing Daxing Maternal and Child Health Care Hospital

续表

辖区 District	医疗机构数 No. of medical institutions	医疗机构名称 Name of medical institutions
大兴区 Daxing	9	国家康复辅具研究中心附属康复医院 Rehabilitation Hospital Affiliated to National Research Center for Rehabilitation Technical Aids
		北京普祥中医肿瘤医院 Beijing Puxiang Traditional Chinese Medicine Cancer Hospital
怀柔区 Huairou	4	北京怀柔医院 Beijing Huairou Hospital
		北京市怀柔区妇幼保健院 Beijing Huairou Maternal and Child Health Care Hospital
		北京市怀柔区中医医院 Beijing Huairou Hospital of Traditional Chinese Medicine
		北京康益德中西医结合肺科医院 Beijing Kangyide Integrated Traditional Chinese and Western Medicine Pulmonary Hospital
平谷区 Pinggu	4	北京市平谷区医院 Beijing Pinggu Hospital
		北京市平谷区中医医院 Beijing Pinggu Hospital of Traditional Chinese Medicine
		北京市平谷区妇幼保健院 Beijing Pinggu Maternal and Child Health Care Hospital
		北京市平谷岳协医院 Beijing Pinggu Yuexie Hospital
密云区 Miyun	3	北京市密云区医院 Beijing Miyun Hospital
		北京市密云区中医医院 Beijing Miyun Hospital of Traditional Chinese Medicine
		北京市密云区妇幼保健院 Beijing Miyun Maternal and Child Health Care Hospital
延庆区 Yanqing	3	北京市延庆区医院（北京大学第三医院延庆医院） Beijing Yanqing Hospital （Peking University Third Hospital Yanqing Hospital）
		北京中医医院延庆医院（北京市延庆区中医医院） Yanqing Hospital of Beijing Chinese Medicine Hospital （Beijing Yanqing Hospital of Traditional Chinese Medicine）
		北京市延庆区妇幼保健院 Beijing Yanqing Maternal and Child Health Care Hospital

2.1.2 北京市肿瘤登记的数据管理及质量控制

肿瘤登记处收集肿瘤病例发病和死亡资料后，需要完成整理分类、查重、死亡补发病、病案核查、随访以及质量控制等环节，才能形成纳入年报分析的数据库。

首先，登记人员在"北京市卫生综合统计信息平台"定期整理医院报告的发病病例信息，根据患者的户籍地址区分本地和外地病例。本地患者纳入数据库，外地患者（约占60%）根据需要转给其他省级登记处。

然后，将当年发病的本地患者按照身份证号码、姓名和出生日期等关键变量与当年发病数据库查重，保存一条信息最全的发病信息，再与往年数据库中近百万病例进行查重。如果未查询到重卡，即按照新增病例统计；若发现重卡，先合并、补充和更新信息，然后再剔除重卡。

将历年的发病数据库与生命统计部门提供的死亡数据库匹配身份证号码，同一患者补充死亡时间和死因；如肿瘤死亡病例在发病数据库查询不到，提示可能存在漏报，此时会及时追溯发病信息并补报。

将当时仍显示存活的现患病例资料发给社区卫生服务中心以开展主动随访工作。登记处定期对存疑的病例开展病案核查工作。

最后，使用国际癌症研究署/国际肿瘤登记协会（International Agency for Research on Cancer/International Association of Cancer

2.1.2 Data management and quality control of the BCR

In order to meet the quality criteria of the data for the Annual Report publishing, after information arrives at the registry, we need to carry out the following steps, including data sort and clean, duplicated cases identification, incident information supplementary using death certification data, re-abstraction and recoding of the cases, active or passive follow-up, and quality control.

Firstly, the registrars, at regular intervals, sorted out the information of the new cases reported by the hospitals on the Beijing Health-care Information Statistical Platform, and distinguished local and non-local cases according to the patient's permanent address. Information of the local patients was included in the database. Data of the non-local patients (about 60% in the reported cases) were transferred to the registries in other provinces as needed.

In order to avoid duplication, the information of new cases diagnosed in the current year was linked to the database of the corresponding year, based on the key variables such as citizen ID number, patient's name, and date of birth. Finally, the most complete entry of information of the patient would be saved, and then re-linked with the database (nearly one million cases) of previous years to find history duplicates. If not matched, the case would be included into the database as a new case of the current year. If the case was identified as duplicated, we would merge, supplement, and update the historic variables of this patient first, and then delete the information of the duplicated one.

The incidence database was linked with the mortality database provided by the vital statistics department by using the number of citizen ID card. We would supplement the date of death and the cause of the death for the same patient if the information from the two databases matched. If the data from the mortality database failed to match with the corresponding incidence data, it indicated that underreporting might have happened, and immediate make-up reporting would follow after tracing the incidence information.

The data and information of the cases recorded as alive in the database would be sent to the community

Registry，IARC/IACR）的肿瘤登记工具软件（Cancer Registry Tools，IARCcrgTools 2.13）中的 Check 程序，逐一检查数据库中所有记录的变量是否完整和有效，同时对不同变量之间是否合乎逻辑进行一致性检查。

2.1.3 北京市肿瘤登记重点工作

2.1.3.1 病案核查

形态学编码为 8000/3、8010/3 的病例，部位不明（O&U）、仅有死亡医学证明书（DCO）和存在逻辑错误的病例，除外淋巴瘤、白血病等极易获取病理诊断的癌种和肝、胆、胰等极难获得病理诊断的癌种，其余病例均需根据病案号返回原报告医院查询病案首页、手术记录、病理报告、检查结果等病历信息，以核实诊断和户籍，补充病理诊断结果，查找肿瘤的具体解剖学部位。每年针对所有的儿童恶性肿瘤资料都开展病案核查，从而对病例进行再摘录和再编码工作。

2.1.3.2 病例随访

随访工作的开展采用被动随访和主动随访相结合的方式进行。肿瘤登记处首先将肿瘤发病库与全死因登记库进行被动匹配。未匹配上的患者再与北京市卫生健康委员会信息统计中心的医院门诊数据库系统匹配身份证号码，1 年之内无门诊和住院记录的患者通过"北京市肿瘤患者随访信息系统"，由社区卫生服务中心 / 站采用电话或者入户的方式定期开展主动随访，获取病例的生存情况。

health service center for active follow-up. And the cancer registry would regularly carry out re-abstraction of medical records for suspected cases.

Finally, the software IARCcrgTools 2.13 provided by the International Agency for Research on Cancer/International Association of Cancer Registry（IARC/IACR）would be used to check whether all the collected variables were complete, accurate, and logically consistent.

2.1.3 Key Tasks of the BCR

2.1.3.1 Medical records re-verification

We would re-verify cases with the codes of 8000/3, 8010/3, O&U and DCO, and those with logical errors, except for cancers that are extremely easy to obtain the pathological diagnosis, such as lymphoma and leukemia, and cancers that are extremely difficult to obtain the pathological diagnosis, such as liver, gallbladder and pancreatic cancer. The cancer registrars would go to the reporting hospital, find the case by the medical record number at the medical record department of the hospital, and re-check the first-page information, surgical records, pathological reports and the findings of examinations and treatment outcomes in the medical records. A further re-verification would focus on whether the patients were local residents or not, their diagnostic and morphological information and the specific anatomical location of the tumor. All children malignant tumors were verified annually by re-extracting and re-coding the information of the medical records.

2.1.3.2 Patient follow-up

Both the passive and the active methods were used to follow the survival status of the patients. The registry's incidence database was linked with the death certificate database for patient identification using their citizen ID card number, then all unmatched cases were re-linked with the cases in the Beijing outpatient service database（within one year）provided by the statistical department of the Beijing Municipal Health Commission. Cases which were still unmatched would be followed-up at the community level by proactive methods, such as telephone calls or home visits.

2.2 北京市肿瘤登记资料收集内容

北京市肿瘤登记处收集北京市户籍人口、常住人口和来京就诊患者中全部恶性肿瘤、原位癌、中枢神经系统良性肿瘤及动态未定肿瘤病例（ICD-10 编码收集范围为 C00-97、D00-09、D32-33、D42-43、D45-47，年报统计范围为北京市户籍人口中编码为 C00-97 和 D45-47 的病例）的发病、死亡和生存状态，以及北京市户籍的相关人口资料。

2.2.1 新发病例资料

个人信息包括姓名、性别、出生日期、年龄、身份证号码、户籍地址、现住址、联系人、联系电话、民族、婚姻状况、职业等。肿瘤信息包括发病日期、解剖学部位（亚部位）、组织学类型、最高诊断依据、肿瘤分期等。转归结局包括是否死亡、死亡日期、死亡原因等。报告单位信息包括报告日期、病案号、报告单位、报告医生等（表 2.2.1）。

2.2 Items of patient information collected by the BCR

The people covered by the data of the BCR include the population of all permanent residents of Beijing, all the people with a Beijing household registration and residents of other provinces who visited Beijing for medical care. The BCR collected the data of new cases, mortality and survival status of the cases diagnosed with malignant tumors, carcinoma in situ, benign tumors of the central nervous system, and dynamic indeterminate tumors （ICD-10 Codes: C00-97, D00-09, D32-33, D42-43, D45-47. Cases with the codes of C00-97, D45-47 and population data of Beijing permanent residents were included into analysis in this annual report）.

2.2.1 Information of new cases

We collected the general information of the new cases, including the name, sex, date of birth, age, ID card number, permanent address, household address, contact person, contact person's telephone number, ethnicity, marital status, occupation; the diagnostic information, including the incidence date, anatomical location（subsite）, histological type, the most valid basis of diagnosis, tumor stage; the outcome information, including the survival status（death or not）, date of death, cause of death; and the information of reporting hospital, including reporting date, medical record number, hospital name, the reporting doctor's name (Table 2.2.1).

表 2.2.1 北京市肿瘤登记数据报告主要内容
Table 2.2.1 Main contents collected by Beijing Cancer Registry

序号 No.	数据采集项 Data collection item	数据类型 Data type	长度 Length	是否必填 If required	备注 Note
01	行政区划代码 Administrative division code	字符 String	6	是 Yes	
02	组织机构代码 Organization code	字符 String	9	是 Yes	各填报单位的组织机构代码 The organization code of each reporting unit
03	机构名称 Organization name	字符 String	200	是 Yes	

续表

序号 No.	数据采集项 Data collection item	数据类型 Data type	长度 Length	是否必填 If required	备注 Note
04	数据年份 Year of data	数字 Numeric	4	是 Yes	
05	数据月份 Month of data	数字 Numeric	2	是 Yes	1 至 12 1 to 12
06	填报人 Reporter's name	字符 String	20	是 Yes	
07	填报日期 Reporting date	日期时间 Date-time	YYYY-MM-DD HH:MM:SS	是 Yes	
08	病案号 Medical record number	字符 String	20	是 Yes	
09	姓名 Name	字符 String	50	是 Yes	
10	性别代码 Sex	字符 String	1	是 Yes	
11	出生日期 Date of birth	日期 Date	YYYY-MM-DD	是 Yes	
12	年龄（岁） Age of diagnosis	数字 Numeric	3	否 No	
13	民族代码 Ethnic group	字符 String	2	否 No	
14	身份证号 Citizen ID card number	字符 String	18	否 No	15 或 18 位 15 or 18 bits
15	婚姻状况代码 Marital status	字符 String	1	是 Yes	
16	户籍省（直辖市、自治区） Household registration province（municipality, autonomous regions）	字符 String	50	否 No	
17	户籍市 Household registration city	字符 String	50	否 No	
18	户籍县 Household registration county	字符 String	50	否 No	

续表

序号 No.	数据采集项 Data collection item	数据类型 Data type	长度 Length	是否必填 If required	备注 Note
19	户籍详细地址 Address of household registration	字符 String	200	肿瘤患者必填 Required for cancer patients	
20	户籍地址区编码 Household registration address district code	字符 String	6	肿瘤患者必填 Required for cancer patients	6 位代码 6 bits
21	户籍地址邮政编码 Household registration address postal code	字符 String	6	否 No	6 位数字 6 bits
22	现住址详细地址（居住半年以上） Current address （living for more than half a year）	字符 String	200	肿瘤患者必填 Required for cancer patients	
23	现住址省（直辖市、自治区） （居住半年以上） Current address province (municipality, autonomous regions) (living for more than half a year)	字符 String	50	否 No	
24	现住址市 Current address city	字符 String	50	否 No	
25	现住址区 Current address district	字符 String	50	否 No	
26	现住址区编码（居住半年以上） Current address district code （living for more than half a year）	字符 String	6	是 Yes	6 位代码 6 bits
27	现住址电话 Phone number	字符 String	20	否 No	
28	现住址邮政编码（居住半年以上） Current address postal code （living for more than half a year）	字符 String	6	否 No	6 位数字 6 bits
29	职业代码 Occupation code	字符 String	2	是 Yes	2 位职业代码 2 bits
30	工作单位及地址 Work unit's name and address	字符 String	200	否 No	
31	联系人姓名 Contact name	字符 String	50	否 No	

续表

序号 No.	数据采集项 Data collection item	数据类型 Data type	长度 Length	是否必填 If required	备注 Note
32	联系人地址 Contact address	字符 String	200	否 No	
33	联系人电话 Contact phone number	字符 String	20	否 No	
34	入院时间 Admission date	日期时间 Date-time	YYYY- MM-DD HH:MM:SS	是 Yes	
35	出院时间 Discharge date	日期时间 Date-time	YYYY- MM-DD HH:MM:SS	是 Yes	
36	出院时主要诊断编码（ICD-10） Main diagnostic code at discharge （ICD-10）	字符 String	30	是 Yes	
37	出院主要诊断名称 Main diagnosis of discharge	字符 String	200	是 Yes	
38	入院病情 Admission condition	字符 String	1	是 Yes	
39	出院时其他诊断编码（ICD-10） Other diagnostic code at discharge （ICD-10）	字符 String	30	是 Yes	
40	出院其他诊断名称 Other diagnosis of discharge	字符 String	200	是 Yes	
41	病理诊断编码（M码） Pathological diagnostic code（M code）	字符 String	50	肿瘤患者必填 Required for cancer patients	
42	病理诊断 Pathological diagnosis	字符 String	100	肿瘤患者必填 Required for cancer patients	
43	最高诊断依据代码 Code of the most valid basis of diagnosis	字符 String	1	肿瘤患者必填 Required for cancer patients	
44	分化程度编码 Differentiation code	字符 String	1	肿瘤患者必填 Required for cancer patients	

续表

序号 No.	数据采集项 Data collection item	数据类型 Data type	长度 Length	是否必填 If required	备注 Note
45	肿瘤分期是否不详 Whether the tumor stage is unknown	字符 String	1	肿瘤患者必填 Required for cancer patients	
46	肿瘤分期 T Stage T	字符 String	1	"肿瘤分期是否不详"填"否"时，此项必填 When filling "No" in "Whether the tumor stage is unknown", "Stage T" is required	
47	肿瘤分期 N Stage N	字符 String	1	"肿瘤分期是否不详"填"否"时，此项必填 When filling "No" in "Whether the tumor stage is unknown", "Stage N" is required	
48	肿瘤分期 M Stage M	字符 String	1	"肿瘤分期是否不详"填"否"时，此项必填 When filling "No" in "Whether the tumor stage is unknown", "Stage M" is required	
49	0~Ⅳ 肿瘤分期 Stage 0~Ⅳ	字符 String	1	"肿瘤分期是否不详"填"否"时，此项必填 When filling "No" in "Whether the tumor stage is unknown", "Stage 0~Ⅳ" is required	
50	主治医师姓名 Name of attending physician	字符 String	20	是 Yes	
51	离院方式代码 Discharge method code	字符 String	1	是 Yes	
52	死亡日期 Date of death	日期 Date	YYYY-MM-DD	否 No	
53	备注 Note	字符 String	500	否 No	

2.2.2 死亡资料

肿瘤死亡资料来源于全人群死因登记报告系统，包括根本死因、间接死因和其他死因涉及肿瘤的死亡资料。除身份证号码、户籍和出生日期等重要的个人信息（用于准确识别患者）外，还应包括死亡日期、死亡年龄、死亡原因主要诊断、诊断级别和依据、死亡地点等。根据填报死亡医学证明书的医院名称和病案号以及填报医生可以进一步追溯发病信息，降低仅有死亡医学证明书的比例（DCO%）。

2.2.3 随访资料

肿瘤病例随访资料包括最后接触时间、生存状态、死亡日期、死亡原因、是否失访、失访原因等。除此之外，北京市肿瘤登记处还对本人病情知晓情况、参加社区健康干预的意愿等进行登记。

2.2.4 人口资料

人口资料来源于北京市公安局逐年公布的人口资料。计算标化率所用的标准人口结构来源于2000年全国人口普查资料和Segi世界标准人口结构。人口资料包括居民人口总数及性别、年龄别人口数或构成。年龄组按小于1岁（0~）、1~4岁（1~）、5~9岁（5~）、10~14岁（10~）……75~79岁（75~）、80~84岁（80~）、85岁及以上（85+）分组。为计算肿瘤相对生存率，还需收集相应年份的寿命表。

2.3 北京市肿瘤登记质量控制指标

北京市肿瘤登记处根据《中国肿瘤登记工作指导手册（2016）》，参照IARC/IACR《五大洲癌症

2.2.2 Mortality data

The cancer mortality data, which included direct cause of death, indirect cause of death and other causes of death related to cancer, were derived from the population-based all causes of death surveillance database. We collected the general information such as patient's citizen ID card number, permanent address, and date of birth, which helped to identify the patient, as well as the date of death, age at death, the main cause of death, the diagnostic basis of death and the place of death. The registrar would track the cases recognized by the death certificates for incidence variables according to the reporting hospital, the number of medical record, and the name of the reporting doctor to reduce the percentage of DCO（DCO%）.

2.2.3 Follow-up data

The data collected through follow-up included date of last contact, survival status, date of death, causes of death, lost to follow-up or not, the reasons of lost to follow-up. In addition, the BCR also registered the patients' awareness of their disease and willingness to participate in community health interventions.

2.2.4 Population data

The population data were derived from the statistics released annually by the Beijing Municipal Public Security Bureau. The standard population structure used to calculate the standardized rate was derived from the 2000 national census data and Segi's world standardized population. The population data included the total number of permanent residents in Beijing and sex- and age- specific number of the population. They are divided into groups by age of 0~, 1~4, 5~9, 10~14··· 75~79, 80~84, 85+. In order to calculate the relative survival of cancer, life tables for the corresponding years were collected.

2.3 Criteria for data quality control

The data quality control criteria of the BCR were made according to the *Chinese Guideline for Cancer Registration（2016）*, and the *Cancer Incidence in Five Continents* volume XI by the International Agency for Research on Cancer（IARC）and International Association of Cancer Registries（IACR）. The

发病率》第XI卷对肿瘤登记质量的有关要求，从数据完整性、有效性和可比性等方面，制定了 MV%、M/I、DCO%、O&U% 等质量控制指标的标准，并且参考北京市历年的报告水平，要求北京市 MV% > 75%、0.50 < M/I < 0.65、DCO% < 2%、O&U% < 10%，并参照此标准开展查漏补缺、病案核查和主动随访工作。

北京市肿瘤登记处在各个环节制定工作规范和质量控制程序并严格执行，质量控制贯穿肿瘤登记工作的全过程。质量控制主要包括四个方面：完整性、有效性、可比性和时效性。

2.3.1 完整性

完整性是指在登记地区目标人群中发现所有发病病例的程度。常用的评价指标有死亡发病比（M/I）、仅有死亡证明书比例（DCO%）、形态学确诊比例（MV%）、病例总数、不同报告来源的比例、每年发病率的稳定性、不同人群发病率的比较、年龄别发病率曲线、儿童肿瘤评价等。

2.3.1.1 死亡发病比（M/I）

死亡发病比是本年度的死亡病例数与发病病例数的比值。M/I 是用于评估肿瘤登记完整性的重要指标。M/I 过低说明存在死亡病例漏报、发病未查重或者随访工作质量差，M/I 过高说明发病存在漏报或者死亡补发病不完整，都与数据的完整性相关。

仅靠所有癌症合计的 M/I 值评估一个地区肿瘤登记的完整性并不准确。例如，我国大部分地区 M/I 介于 0.6~0.8 之间，但是北京市生存率较高的甲状腺癌和乳腺癌患者所占比例大，就会拉低死亡病

completeness, validity and comparability of the data were evaluated using indicators such as MV%, M/I, DCO%, and O&U%. After taking the historical quality control data at BCR into consideration, the corresponding cutoff values and criteria for the indicators were set (MV% > 75%, 0.50 < M/I < 0.65, DCO% < 2% and O&U% < 10%). The BCR carried out the quality control, re-abstraction of medical records and proactive follow-up based on the above criteria.

The BCR strictly implemented the guidelines and quality control procedures it had established in all processes. The quality control focused on four aspects: completeness, validity, comparability, and timeliness.

2.3.1 Completeness

The completeness of cancer registry data concerns about to what extent the new cases occurred in a defined population were registered in the cancer registration database. The indicators to evaluate the completeness includes the M/I, DCO%, MV%, the total number of registrations, the proportions of cases by reported sources, year-on-year incidence rate growth, population-specific data, age-specific data, and the incidence of childhood cancers and its year-on-year change.

2.3.1.1 Mortality to incidence ratio （M/I）

The M/I refers to the ratio of the number of deaths to the number of new cases in the current year. It is an important indicator for the assessment of the completeness of cancer registration data. If the M/I is too low, it indicates that the deaths may have been underreported, duplicated newly diagnosed cases exist, or the quality of follow-up is poor; if the M/I is too high, it indicates that some new cases may have been underreported or there is incomplete recognition and supplementation of cases by death certificate.

It is not a good choice to evaluate the completeness of cancer data in a defined region based on the M/I value of all cancers. For example, the M/I of most areas in China was between 0.6 and 0.8. However, the M/I of all cancers in Beijing was less than 0.55 due to the higher proportion of the patients with thyroid and breast cancers, both having a higher survival rate. Therefore,

例数，使 M/I 的比值不足 0.55，因此评估单癌种的 M/I 更为合理。

it is more reasonable to evaluate the M/I of an individual cancer in a defined population.

2.3.1.2 仅有死亡医学证明书比例（DCO%）

DCO% 是指仅有死亡医学证明书的病例占所有癌症发病病例的比例，意味着患者生前没有肿瘤的诊疗记录或者无法获得诊疗信息，更不可能有形态学确诊的结果，病例的发病日期即为死亡日期。死亡医学证明书是发现恶性肿瘤病例的有效补充途径，DCO% 也是间接评价由死亡医学证明书发现病例比例（DCN%）的指标。DCO 病例是 DCN 追溯流程完成后的剩余部分，DCO% 理论上应维持在一个恒定的较低水平，但不能为零。DCO% 是评价一个地区肿瘤登记资料完整性的重要指标。该指标过低，提示死亡补发病工作流程有误，未经治疗或者异地治疗的恶性肿瘤死亡病例未被补充到发病数据库中，存在漏报；DCO% 过高，则提示死亡病例未有效追溯发病信息，发病数据缺乏完整性。

2.3.1.3 形态学确诊比例（MV%）

形态学确诊（morphological verification, MV）的比例包括病理诊断和细胞学 / 血片诊断的病例所占百分比，既是完整性的指标，又是有效性的一个重要指标。IACR 建议 MV% > 75%。但是该指标并不是越高越好，过高的 MV% 说明病例均来源于医院报告，其他报告渠道可能存在漏报；过低的 MV% 可能是未及时获取病理报告造成的，也可能是因为某一不易获取病理诊断的癌种（例如肝癌）在所有癌种中占比较高所致，影响了数据的完整性。

2.3.1.2 Proportion of cases recognized by death certificate only （DCO%）

The DCO% refers to the proportion of cases with death certificate only in all cancer cases, which means that the diagnosis and treatment information, such as the morphological type, was not available and the incidence date of the case is the same as the date of death. The death certification is an effective supplementation to find cancer cases, and DCO% is also an indicator that could be used for indirect evaluation of the proportion of cases first notified by death certificate（DCN%）. DCO cases are the remainder of cases after the identification of the new cases retrospectively by death certificate（DCN）. Theoretically, the DCO% should be maintained in a constantly lower level, but not zero. DCO% is an important indicator for evaluating the completeness of cancer registration data in a defined region. If DCO% is too low, it indicates that there might be problems in the process of identification of cases by death certificate: the cases that received diagnosis and treatment in outpatient departments or received treatment out of the registration region were underreported or omitted. A too high DCO% means that the incidence information of death cases was not effectively traced, and the incidence information was not fully supplemented.

2.3.1.3 Proportion of morphological verified cases （MV%）

The MV% refers to the percentage of cases diagnosed by pathology or cytology/hematology. It is an important indicator of both completeness and validity of cancer registration data. The cutoff value of the MV% that IACR recommended was > 75%. However, it's not the higher the better for this value. If the MV% is too high, it may indicate that the cases are all reported by hospitals, and there may be underreporting with the other reporting sources; if the MV% is too low, it may indicate that the results of the pathology were not reported in time. Another explanation for the excessively low MV% is that a relatively high proportion of a certain type of cancer which is difficult to obtain pathology（such as liver cancer）accounts for an excessively high proportion in all the cases, which also affects the completeness of the data.

$$MV\% = \frac{\text{最高诊断依据为 5、6、7、8 的例数}^{①}}{\text{报告肿瘤病例总例数}} \times 100\%$$

$$MV\% = \frac{\text{The number of the patients with the most valid basis of diagnosis 5, 6, 7, 8}^{②}}{\text{The total number of the patients}} \times 100\%$$

2.3.1.4 身份证号码的填写比例

鉴于肿瘤登记工作中复诊和随访的信息追溯都需要身份证号码作为关键变量，因此北京市非常重视身份证信息的收集和质控，医院上传的病例都需要校验身份证号码才能通过。近年，北京市肿瘤病例身份证号码的填写率均超过 99%。

2.3.2 有效性

有效性是指登记病例中具有给定特征（例如肿瘤部位、年龄、性别、诊断和编码）真正属性的病例所占的比例。再摘录与再编码方法是评价有效性最客观的方法，即通过再摘录与再编码核对符合程度以评估既往采集信息的准确率。

常用的评价指标有部位不明比例（O&U%）、形态学确诊比例（MV%）和仅有死亡医学证明书比例（DCO%）。为保障有效性，北京市肿瘤登记处定期对身份证号码、出生日期、性别、继发或不明部位，以及无组织学诊断的病例开展病案记录核对、再摘录和再编码。

2.3.2.1 部位不明比例（O&U%）

肿瘤登记资料的有效性受错误和缺失资料的影响。同时，由于受临床诊疗水平及患者依从性的客

2.3.1.4 Proportion of cases that had filled in citizen ID card number

In view of the fact that the citizen ID card number is required as a key variable for re-abstraction of medical records and the follow-up, the BCR made great efforts to ensure the quality control of ID card number, which would help improve the completeness of data. The citizen ID card number of all cancer cases uploaded to the on-line reporting system by hospitals needed to be verified. The proportion of cases that had filled in the numbers among the diagnosed cancer cases was more than 99% in recent years in Beijing.

2.3.2 Validity

The validity refers to the proportion of registered cases with real attributes of a given characteristic (such as tumor location, age, sex, diagnosis, and code). In other words, to assess the accuracy of previously collected information and check the degree of conformity, re-extracting and re-coding would be conducted.

Commonly used evaluation indicators are O&U%, DCO%, and MV%. To ensure the accuracy, the BCR regularly re-extracts and re-codes the information of the patients, such as citizen ID card number, date of birth, sex, metastatic or unknown tumor sites, and cases without histological diagnosis.

2.3.2.1 Proportion of cases of other or unspecified sites (O&U%)

The validity of cancer registration data is affected by reporting errors and missing items. At the same time, due to the doctor's clinical diagnosis and treatment capacity and patient compliance, the BCR would

---

① 5，细胞学和血片；6，病理（继发）；7，病理（原发）；8，尸检（有病理）。

② 5，cytology or hematology；6，histology of metastasis；7，histology of primary；8，autopsy with concurrent or previous histology.

观影响，每年北京市肿瘤登记处都会收到继发病例和原发部位不详病例的报告，但历年的 O&U% 应该维持在相对较低的水平。

$$O\&U\% = \frac{C26 + C39 + C48 + C76\text{-}80 + C97 \text{ 的例数}^{①}}{\text{报告肿瘤病例总例数}} \times 100\%$$

2.3.2.2 形态学确诊比例（MV%）

MV% 是衡量数据有效性的一个重要指标。过低的 MV% 意味着大量的病例未经形态学诊断的确认，仅靠临床和影像等方式诊断，不排除有误诊病例混入的可能性。而且未经病理分型的病例资料，对其病因和预后因素开展分析非常局限，会影响干预措施和卫生政策的制定，失去了肿瘤登记的目的和意义。

但是不同恶性肿瘤获取病理结果的难易程度不同，MV% 需要分癌种进行评估。例如肝癌和胰腺癌，由于病程短，发现时多数患者失去手术机会，其所在的解剖学位置也不易进行穿刺，因此 MV% 通常只有 20%～30%；相反，消化道的恶性肿瘤能通过内镜活检直接获得病理结果，MV% 高达 99% 以上。因此，评估数据库的准确性不要局限于总体癌症的 MV%。

receive the reports of the cases with metastasis or cases with unspecified primary sites each year. Ideally, the O&U% should be maintained at a relatively low level in a defined region.

$$O\&U\% = \frac{\text{The number of cases with the codes of}}{\text{C26 + C39 + C48 + C76-80 + C97}^{②}} \times 100\%$$

2.3.2.2 Proportion of morphological verified cases （MV%）

The MV% is an important indicator to measure the validity of the data. If the MV% is too low, it means that a large number of cases were not confirmed by microscopic diagnosis, and were confirmed by clinical and imaging evidence only, which increases the possibility of inaccurate diagnosis. Moreover, if a database included many cancer cases that were confirmed by non-microscopic evidence, it would hamper the researchers to explore the etiology and prognostic factors of cancer cases and mislead the health policy makers when they were to establish the intervention measures and health policies. In that case, cancer registration would become meaningless.

Nevertheless, the availability of pathological results for different tumors is quite different, so the MV% needs to be assessed by specific cancer sites. For example, for liver and pancreatic cancers, due to the short course of disease, most patients would lose the opportunity for surgery when they were diagnosed, complicated by the difficulty for centesis due to the anatomical location of the organs, the MV% would stand at 20%-30%; on the contrary, tissues from the digestive tract can be biopsied easily by endoscopy, therefore, the MV% of digestive tract tumors would stand as high as 99% and above. So, the accuracy of the data should not be evaluated by the MV% value of all the cancer sites. Instead, the value of specific cancer sites should be used for the evaluation.

---

① C26、C39、C48、C76-80 和 C97 均为 ICD-10 编码。C26，其他和不明确的消化系统恶性肿瘤；C39，呼吸和胸腔内器官的恶性肿瘤；C48，腹膜后和腹膜恶性肿瘤；C76-80，不明确、继发和未特指部位的恶性肿瘤；C97，独立的多个部位原发恶性肿瘤。

② ICD-10: C26, Malignant neoplasm of other and ill-defined digestive organs; C39, Malignant neoplasm of other and ill-defined sites in the respiratory system and intrathoracic organs; C48, Retroperitoneal and peritoneal malignancies; C76-80, Malignant neoplasms of ill-defined, secondary and unspecified sites; C97, Malignant neoplasms of independent（primary）multiple sites.

2.3.2.3 仅有死亡医学证明书比例（DCO%）

DCO% 是有效性的一个负面指标。DCO 意味着无法获取形态学诊断，因此 DCO% 过高会引起较低的 MV%，资料的有效性较差。但是前面也提到，由于客观条件的限制，DCO 无法避免，因此需要辩证地看待。此外，DCO% 过低也是不可信的。

2.3.3 可比性

数据结果可比的基本先决条件是采用通用的标准或定义。通常而言，可比性是指发病率间的不同不是因为各登记处之间的统计标准或数据质量不同而产生的。可比性涉及以下几个指标：对"发病"的定义，对原发、复发和转移的诊断标准，分类与编码，死亡证明等。

2.3.3.1 外部一致性

北京市肿瘤登记处所收集资料中的肿瘤部位编码采用 ICD-10 编码，形态学编码采用《国际疾病分类肿瘤学专辑》（第 2 版）（*International Classification of Diseases for Oncology, 2nd Revision*, ICD-O-2）编码，整理过程中增加一列《国际疾病分类肿瘤学专辑》（第 3 版）（*International Classification of Diseases for Oncology, 3rd Revision*, ICD-O-3）编码。发病日期统一选择首次住院日期，多原发恶性肿瘤的判定采用 IARC 标准。中国标准人口年龄结构采用 2000 年全国人口普查资料，世界标准人口年龄结构采用 Segi 世界标准人口构成。

因此，比较各地区的恶性肿瘤发病、死亡和生存水平不应仅限报表数据的简单对比，还要结合该地区编码种类、病例收集范围、发病时间定义、多原发恶性肿瘤判断标准、标准人口结构等影响因素综合判断。

2.3.2.3 Proportion of cases recognized by death certificate only （DCO%）

The DCO% is a negative indicator of validity. DCO means that no information of morphological diagnosis has been collected. Therefore, a remarkably high DCO% will cause a lower MV%, and poor validity of the data. However, it has been mentioned earlier in the report that DCO cannot be avoided and should be viewed dialectically. If the DCO% is too low, it is unreliable too.

2.3.3 Comparability

The basic prerequisite for comparability of cancer registry data is the use of uniform standards or definitions. Generally speaking, comparability means that the difference in incidence rates in different regions or countries is not due to differences in statistical standards or data quality among the population-based registries. Comparability involves the following indicators: definition of "incidence"; diagnostic criteria for primary, recurrent and metastatic diseases; classification and coding; and death certificate, etc.

2.3.3.1 External Consistency

The coding of cancer site in the BCR uses the ICD-10, and the morphological coding uses the ICD-O-2 (*International Classification of Diseases for Oncology, 2nd Revision*). A new code, the ICD-O-3 (*International Classification of Diseases for Oncology, 3rd Revision*) coding, which was transformed from ICD-O-2, was added in the process of data cleaning. The incidence date was defined as the date of first hospitalization, and the criteria of recognizing multiple primary malignancies was adopted using IARC standards. For Chinese standard age structure, we used the 2000 National Census data; and for the world's standard age structure, Segi's structure of the world population was used.

Therefore, comparison of the incidence, death, and survival levels of cancer cases in various regions should not be limited to simple comparison of the data reported in the Annual Reports, but should take the influencing factors into consideration. These factors include the coding method, cases inclusion and exclusion criteria, definition of the incidence date, multiple primary tumor criteria, and standard age structure in the region.

2.3.3.2 内部一致性

随访患者无准确死亡日期的，登记到某年的记录为当年 7 月 1 日，登记到某月的按 15 日登记。逻辑校验采用北京市报告系统自带的逻辑校验和有效性校验功能，包括年龄 / 出生日期、身份证有效性、性别 / 部位、性别 / 形态学、部位 / 形态学、最高诊断依据和形态学诊断的逻辑错误，日期一致性（死亡日期和随访日期不得早于发病日期、死亡日期不得早于最后随访日期等），编码一致性（发病编码和死亡编码的匹配）等，最后采用 IARCcrgTools 2.13 软件中的 Check 程序，对数据库病例逐一做最终检查。

2.3.4 时效性

时效性指肿瘤登记处收集、处理和发布完整及准确的肿瘤登记资料的及时性，一般指发病日期（诊断日期）到数据被利用时（年报、研究报告、政府发布、论文）的时间间隔。北京市各医院在患者出院 1 个月内报告病例资料，登记处需要等待 1 年完善患者的治疗及病理诊断结果。北京市疾病预防控制中心每年初提供上一年度的死亡病例数据库，登记处匹配死亡信息作为发病数据漏报的补充。由于大部分癌症患者的生存时间为 1~3 年，因此死亡补发病工作持续 3 年才能补充完整；3 年期间每年定期随访患者，至少完成 1 次病案核查工作。

为了保证数据的完整性和有效性，需要留给登记处足够的时间核实和补充资料。根据 IARC/IACR 的建议，全球各个国家和地区的肿瘤登记处通常于诊断年份后的 3 年发布数据。

2.3.3.2 Internal consistency

If a patient was followed up, but only the accurate death year was available, the deceased date of this patient would be recorded as July 1st, and if both the death year and month were available, the deceased date of the patient would be recorded as the 15th of the month. The logic verification process used the logic and validity check function of the BCR's reporting system. The verified contents included age/birth date, citizen ID validity, sex/tumor location, sex/morphology, tumor location/morphology, most valid basis of diagnosis and morphology diagnosis, date consistency (death date and follow-up date should not be earlier than incidence date, death date should not be earlier than last follow-up date, etc.), coding consistency (incidence code and death code matched or not), etc.; and a final check of all cases was performed using the software of IARCcrgTools 2.13.

2.3.4 Timeliness

Timeliness refers to the rapidity at which a registry can collect, finish quality control and publish reliable and complete cancer data. Generally, it refers to the time interval from the incidence date (date of first diagnosis) to the time when the data is used (for annual reports, government releases, and research papers). Hospitals in Beijing would submit the information of new cancer cases within one month after the patient was discharged. The registry would need one year to do the quality control of the patient's treatment and pathological diagnosis results; the Beijing Center for Disease Prevention and Control would provide the data of all cases of death of the previous year at the beginning of each year, and the BCR would link to this mortality database, using it as a supplementary source to detect the underreported cases. Since the survival time of most cancer patients was between 1-3 years, the supplementation could only be completed after 3 years, which would help the BCR to meet the criteria of completeness of cancer registration data; patients were followed up regularly every year during the above mentioned 3 years, and at least one medical record verification should be completed during the quality control period.

In order to ensure the completeness and validity of the data, it is necessary to leave enough time for cancer registries to verify and supplement the information. According to the recommendations of IARC/IACR, the registries around the world usually release data three years after the diagnosis year.

2.4 本肿瘤登记年报质量控制评价

2019 年，北京市肿瘤登记数据库的形态学确诊比例（MV%）为 80.89%，仅有死亡医学证明书比例（DCO%）为 0.05%，死亡/发病比（M/I）为 0.47，部位不明比例（O&U%）为 1.32%（表 2.4.1）。

2.4 Data quality control of this annual report

The MV%, DCO%, M/I and O&U% of the cancer cases included for analysis in this annual report were 80.89%, 0.05%, 0.47 and 1.32%, respectively, in Beijing in 2019 (Table 2.4.1) .

（撰稿 王宁，校稿 杨雷）

表 2.4.1 2019 年北京市肿瘤登记数据质量控制评价结果一览表
Table 2.4.1 Quality indicators of the cancer data in Beijing, 2019

部位 Site	全市 All areas			城区 Urban areas			郊区 Peri-urban areas		
	MV%	DCO%	M/I	MV%	DCO%	M/I	MV%	DCO%	M/I
口腔和咽 Oral cavity & pharynx	82.05	0.00	0.47	81.73	0.00	0.45	82.77	0.00	0.52
鼻咽 Nasopharynx	66.67	0.00	0.95	69.23	0.00	0.89	60.71	0.00	1.07
食管 Esophagus	61.51	0.00	0.85	61.72	0.00	0.85	61.27	0.00	0.84
胃 Stomach	72.60	0.01	0.72	74.39	0.01	0.72	68.68	0.01	0.74
结直肠 Colon-rectum	86.61	0.00	0.43	86.06	0.01	0.45	87.75	0.00	0.40
肝 Liver	37.40	0.02	0.82	41.48	0.02	0.82	31.40	0.01	0.83
胆囊 Gallbladder	49.35	0.00	0.83	48.85	0.00	0.83	50.10	0.00	0.83
胰腺 Pancreas	36.57	0.00	0.92	37.51	0.00	0.93	34.44	0.00	0.89
喉 Larynx	84.64	0.00	0.45	87.10	0.00	0.45	81.20	0.00	0.46
肺 Lung	71.45	0.01	0.62	73.65	0.02	0.60	67.67	0.00	0.65
其他胸腔器官 Other thoracic organs	80.63	0.00	0.68	80.73	0.00	0.71	80.39	0.00	0.61

续表

部位 Site	全市 All areas			城区 Urban areas			郊区 Peri-urban areas		
	MV%	DCO%	M/I	MV%	DCO%	M/I	MV%	DCO%	M/I
骨 Bone	69.93	0.00	0.61	67.86	0.00	0.67	72.46	0.00	0.55
皮肤（黑色素瘤） Skin（Melanoma）	100.00	0.00	0.55	100.00	0.00	0.62	100.00	0.00	0.41
女性乳腺 Female breast	95.94	0.00	0.20	95.85	0.00	0.21	96.13	0.00	0.16
子宫颈 Cervix	85.58	0.00	0.37	88.06	0.00	0.36	81.71	0.00	0.39
子宫体 Uterus	96.19	0.00	0.16	96.52	0.00	0.17	95.60	0.00	0.14
卵巢 Ovary	86.13	0.00	0.57	84.97	0.00	0.58	88.36	0.00	0.55
前列腺 Prostate	88.15	0.00	0.39	88.86	0.00	0.39	86.12	0.00	0.38
睾丸 Testis	95.74	0.00	0.15	93.75	0.00	0.19	100.00	0.00	0.07
肾 Kidney	87.98	0.00	0.33	88.45	0.00	0.35	86.95	0.00	0.27
膀胱 Bladder	88.66	0.00	0.39	88.46	0.00	0.40	89.06	0.00	0.37
脑 Brain	78.46	0.00	0.72	81.80	0.00	0.67	72.06	0.00	0.82
甲状腺 Thyroid	99.17	0.00	0.02	99.37	0.00	0.02	98.82	0.00	0.02
淋巴瘤 Lymphoma	99.70	0.00	0.61	99.82	0.00	0.63	99.45	0.00	0.58
白血病 Leukemia	100.00	0.00	0.74	100.00	0.00	0.81	100.00	0.00	0.64
其他 Others	80.51	0.01	0.46	79.47	0.01	0.48	82.53	0.01	0.41
合计 **All sites**	80.89	0.05	0.47	81.96	0.06	0.47	78.87	0.04	0.47

3 统计分类指标释义
Interpretation of Statistical Items Classification

3.1 统计分类

3.1.1 癌症分类

参照国际上常用的癌症 ICD-10 分类统计表，根据 ICD-10 "C" 类编码的前三位，将癌症细分类为 59 个部位、26 大类。真性红细胞增多症（D45）、骨髓增生异常综合征（D46）、淋巴造血和有关组织动态未定肿瘤（D47）归入髓样白血病。详见表 3.1.1 和表 3.1.2。

3.1 Items classification

3.1.1 Cancer classification

Based on the ICD-10 classification principles, neoplasms were subdivided into 59 main sites, correspondent to 26 categories according to the first three number of the "C" codes. Polycythemia vera（D45）, myelodysplastic syndrome（D46）and lymphoid, hematopoietic, and related tissue tumors with uncertain behavior（D47）were classified as myeloid leukemia in data analysis. See Table 3.1.1 and Table 3.1.2 for details.

表 3.1.1 常用癌症分类统计表（细分类）
Table 3.1.1 Detailed cancer classification of ICD-10

序号 No.	部位 Site	ICD-10
1	唇 Lip	C00
2	舌 Tongue	C01-02
3	口 Mouth	C03-06
4	唾液腺 Salivary glands	C07-08
5	扁桃体 Tonsil	C09
6	其他口咽 Other oropharynx	C10
7	鼻咽 Nasopharynx	C11
8	下咽 Hypopharynx	C12-13
9	咽，部位不明 Pharynx unspecified	C14
10	食管 Esophagus	C15
11	胃 Stomach	C16
12	小肠 Small intestine	C17
13	结肠 Colon	C18

续表

序号 No.	部位 Site	ICD-10
14	直肠 Rectum	C19-20
15	肛门 Anus	C21
16	肝 Liver	C22
17	胆囊及其他 Gallbladder etc.	C23-24
18	胰腺 Pancreas	C25
19	鼻、鼻窦及其他 Nose, sinuses etc.	C30-31
20	喉 Larynx	C32
21	气管、支气管、肺 Trachea, bronchus & lung	C33-34
22	其他胸腔器官 Other thoracic organs	C37-38
23	骨 Bone	C40-41
24	皮肤（黑色素瘤） Skin（melanoma）	C43
25	皮肤（其他） Skin（other）	C44
26	间皮瘤 Mesothelioma	C45
27	卡波西肉瘤 Kaposi sarcoma	C46
28	周围神经、其他结缔组织和软组织 Peripheral nerves, other connective & soft tissue	C47, C49
29	乳腺 Breast	C50
30	外阴 Vulva	C51
31	阴道 Vagina	C52
32	子宫颈 Cervix uteri	C53
33	子宫体 Corpus uteri	C54
34	子宫，部位不明 Uterus unspecified	C55
35	卵巢 Ovary	C56
36	其他女性生殖器 Other female genital organs	C57
37	胎盘 Placenta	C58
38	阴茎 Penis	C60
39	前列腺 Prostate	C61
40	睾丸 Testis	C62
41	其他男性生殖器 Other male genital organs	C63

续表

序号 No.	部位 Site	ICD-10
42	肾 Kidney	C64
43	肾盂 Renal pelvis	C65
44	输尿管 Ureter	C66
45	膀胱 Bladder	C67
46	其他泌尿器官 Other urinary organs	C68
47	眼 Eye	C69
48	脑、神经系统 Brain, nervous system	C70-72
49	甲状腺 Thyroid	C73
50	肾上腺 Adrenal gland	C74
51	其他内分泌腺 Other endocrine	C75
52	霍奇金淋巴瘤 Hodgkin lymphoma	C81
53	非霍奇金淋巴瘤 Non-Hodgkin lymphoma	C82-85, C96
54	免疫增生性疾病 Immunoproliferative diseases	C88
55	多发性骨髓瘤 Multiple myeloma	C90
56	淋巴样白血病 Lymphoid leukemia	C91
57	髓样白血病 Myeloid leukemia	C92-94, D45-47
58	白血病，未特指 Leukemia unspecified	C95
59	其他或未指明部位 Other and unspecified（O&U）	C26,C39,C48,C76-80,C97
	所有部位合计 All sites	C00-97, D45-47
	所有部位除外 C44 All sites except C44	C00-97, D45-47 exc. C44

表 3.1.2 常用癌症分类统计表（大分类）
Table 3.1.2 Broad cancer classification of ICD-10

序号 No.	部位全称 Full name of site	部位简称 Short name of site	ICD-10
1	口腔和咽喉（除外鼻咽） Oral cavity & pharynx exc. nasopharynx	口腔和咽 Oral cavity & pharynx	C00-10, C12-14
2	鼻咽 Nasopharynx	鼻咽 Nasopharynx	C11
3	食管 Esophagus	食管 Esophagus	C15

续表

序号 No.	部位全称 Full name of site	部位简称 Short name of site	ICD-10
4	胃 Stomach	胃 Stomach	C16
5	结肠、直肠和肛门 Colon, rectum & anus	结直肠 Colon-rectum	C18-21
6	肝 Liver	肝 Liver	C22
7	胆囊及其他 Gallbladder and others	胆囊 Gallbladder	C23-24
8	胰腺 Pancreas	胰腺 Pancreas	C25
9	喉 Larynx	喉 Larynx	C32
10	气管、支气管和肺 Trachea, bronchus & lung	肺 Lung	C33-34
11	其他胸腔器官 Other thoracic organs	其他胸腔器官 Other thoracic organs	C37-38
12	骨 Bone	骨 Bone	C40-41
13	皮肤黑色素瘤 Melanoma of skin	皮肤黑色素瘤 Melanoma of skin	C43
14	乳腺 Breast	乳腺 Breast	C50
15	子宫颈 Cervix uteri	子宫颈 Cervix	C53
16	子宫体及子宫部位不明 Uterus & unspecified	子宫体 Uterus	C54-55
17	卵巢 Ovary	卵巢 Ovary	C56
18	前列腺 Prostate	前列腺 Prostate	C61
19	睾丸 Testis	睾丸 Testis	C62
20	肾及泌尿系统部位不明 Kidney & unspecified urinary organs	肾 Kidney	C64-66, C68
21	膀胱 Bladder	膀胱 Bladder	C67
22	脑、神经系统 Brain, nervous system	脑 Brain	C70-C72
23	甲状腺 Thyroid	甲状腺 Thyroid	C73
24	淋巴瘤 Lymphoma	淋巴瘤 Lymphoma	C81-85, C88, C90, C96
25	白血病 Leukemia	白血病 Leukemia	C91-95, D45-47
26	其他或未指明部位 Other and unspecified	其他或未指明部位（O&U）	C26,C39,C48,C76-80,C97
	所有部位合计 All sites	合计 All sites	C00-97, D45-47

3.1.2 地区分类

城区包括东城、西城、朝阳、海淀、丰台、石景山，郊区包括门头沟、房山、通州、顺义、昌平、大兴、怀柔、平谷、密云、延庆。

3.2 常用统计指标

3.2.1 年均人口数

年均人口数是计算发病（死亡）率指标的分母，精确算法是一年内每一天暴露于发病（死亡）危险的生存人数之和除以年内天数，但实际上很难掌握每一天的生存人数，因而常用年初和年末人口数的算术平均数作为年均人口数的近似值。

$$\text{年均人口数（人）} = \frac{\text{年初（上年末）人口数} + \text{年末人口数}}{2}$$

年中人口数指 7 月 1 日零时人口数。如果人口数变化均匀，年中人口数等于年均人口数，可以用年中人口数代替年均人口数。

3.2.2 性别、年龄别人口数

根据北京市公安局年末提供的户籍人口分性别百岁表计算。年龄的分组规定除 0 岁组和 1~4 岁组以外，以间隔 5 岁为一组，即 0~、1~4、5~9、10~14…75~79、80~84、85+，共计 19 组。

3.2.3 发病（死亡）率

发病（死亡）率又称为粗发病（死亡）率，是反映人口发病（死亡）情况最基本的指标，是指某年该地登记的每 10 万人口癌症新发（死亡）病例

3.1.2 Area classification

The urban areas of Beijing include Dongcheng, Xicheng, Chaoyang, Haidian, Fengtai, and Shijingshan; and the peri-urban areas include Mentougou, Fangshan, Tongzhou, Shunyi, Changping, Daxing, Huairou, Pinggu, Miyun, and Yanqing.

3.2 Statistical indicators

3.2.1 Average annual population

Average annual population is the denominator used in the calculation of the incidence（mortality）rates. Its theoretical value is the number of persons at risk of incidence（death）each day in a specific year divided by number of the days in the year. Considering the complexity of such calculation, we would often use the estimation/calculation as expressed by the following formula:

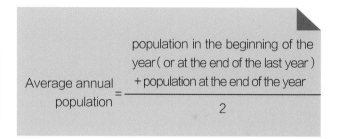

The number of mid-year population refers to the number of the population at 00:00 on July 1st. If the number of the population is relatively stable, the mid-year population could be used to represent average annual population.

3.2.2 Sex- and age-specific population

The sex- and age-specific population is provided by the Beijing Municipal Public Security Bureau. People were divided into 19 age groups of 0-, 1-4, 5-9, 10-14… 75-79, 80-84, 85+years, respectively.

3.2.3 Incidence（mortality）rate

The incidence（mortality）rate is a measure of the frequency at which an event, such as a new case of cancer（cancer death）, occurs in a population over a period of time.

数，反映人口发病（死亡）水平。

$$发病（死亡）率（1/10\ 万）= \frac{某年某地癌症新病例（死亡）数}{某年某地年均人口数} \times 100\ 000$$

3.2.4 性别、年龄别发病（死亡）率

性别和年龄结构是影响恶性肿瘤发病（死亡）水平的重要因素，性别、年龄别发病（死亡）率是统计研究的重要指标。

$$某性别（年龄别）发病（死亡）率（1/10\ 万）= \frac{某性别（年龄组）发病（死亡）人数}{同性别（年龄组）人口数} \times 100\ 000$$

3.2.5 年龄调整率（标化率）

由于粗发病（死亡）率受人口年龄构成的影响较大，因此在对比分析不同地区的发病（死亡）率或同一地区人群不同时期的发病（死亡）水平时，为消除人口年龄结构对发病（死亡）水平的影响，需要计算按年龄标准化的发病（死亡）率，即按照某一标准人口的年龄结构所计算的发病（死亡）率。本年报采用的中国标准人口是 2000 年全国第五次人口普查的人口构成（以此计算的标化率简称中标率），世界标准人口采用 Segi 标准人口构成（以此计算的标化率简称世标率）。表 3.2.1 为中国 2000 年人口结构和 Segi 世界标准人口年龄构成，可供计算年龄标准化率时选用。

$$Incidence（mortality）rate\ per\ 100{,}000\ pyrs = \frac{\begin{array}{c}No.\ of\ new\ cases（new\ deaths）\\ arising\ in\ a\ defined\ population\ in\ a\\ specific\ period\ of\ time\end{array}}{\begin{array}{c}Total\ person\text{-}years\ at\ risk\ in\ that\\ population\ during\ that\ period\ of\ time\end{array}} \times 100{,}000$$

3.2.4 Sex- and age-specific incidence （mortality）rates

Sex and age structure are important factors influencing the cancer incidence and mortality. Sex- and age-specific rates are important statistical indicators in cancer epidemiology.

$$Sex\text{-}\ or\ age\text{-}specific\ incidence（mortality）rate\ per\ 100{,}000\ pyrs = \frac{\begin{array}{c}No.\ of\ new\ cases\ arising\ in\ a\ certain\\ sex\ or\ age\ group\ in\ a\ defined\ population\\ and\ in\ a\ specific\ period\ of\ time\end{array}}{\begin{array}{c}Person\text{-}years\ at\ risk\ in\ that\ sex\ or\\ age\ group\ in\ the\ same\ population\\ and\ during\ that\ period\ of\ time\end{array}} \times 100{,}000$$

3.2.5 Age standardized rates （ASRs）

Because the crude incidence（mortality）rate would be substantially affected by the age structure of the population, when comparing the incidence（mortality）rate in different regions or in the same region but at different periods of time, in order to eliminate the influence of the population's age structure on the incidence or mortality, it is necessary to calculate the age-standardized incidence（mortality）rate（ASIR or ASMR）. In other words, the ASIR or ASMR represents the incidence or mortality rate after adjusting of age by a standardized age structure of a certain population. The Chinese standard population used in this annual report adopts the age structure of the fifth national census in 2000, and the world standard population adopts Segi's standard population structure. Table 3.2.1 shows the age structures of the Chinese and the world standard population, which could be used when calculating the age-standardized rates.

表 3.2.1 标准人口构成
Table 3.2.1 Standard population

年龄组（岁） Age group（years）	中国人口构成（2000 年） Number of persons in Chinese standard population（2000）	Segi 世界标准人口构成 Number of persons in Segi's population
0~	13 793 799	2 400
1~4	55 184 575	9 600
5~9	90 152 587	10 000
10~14	125 396 633	9 000
15~19	103 031 165	9 000
20~24	94 573 174	8 000
25~29	117 602 265	8 000
30~34	127 314 298	6 000
35~39	109 147 295	6 000
40~44	81 242 945	6 000
45~49	85 521 045	6 000
50~54	63 304 200	5 000
55~59	46 370 375	4 000
60~64	41 703 848	4 000
65~69	34 780 460	3 000
70~74	25 574 149	2 000
75~79	15 928 330	1000
80~84	7 989 158	500
85+	4 001 925	500
合计 Total	1 242 612 226	100 000

年龄标化发病（死亡）率的计算（直接法）：

（1）计算年龄组发病（死亡）率。

（2）以各年龄组发病（死亡）率乘以相应的标准人口年龄构成百分比，得到相应的理论发病（死亡）率。

（3）各年龄组的理论发病（死亡）率相加之和即为年龄标化发病（死亡）率。

$$标化发病（死亡）率（1/10万）= \frac{\Sigma[标准人口各年龄组人口数或构成比 \times 年龄别发病（死亡）率]}{\Sigma标准人口各年龄组人口数或构成比} \times 100\,000$$

3.2.6 分类构成比

各类恶性肿瘤发病（死亡）构成比可以反映各类恶性肿瘤对居民健康危害的情况。恶性肿瘤发病（死亡）分类构成比的计算公式如下：

$$某恶性肿瘤构成比（\%）= \frac{某恶性肿瘤发病（死亡）人数}{恶性肿瘤总发病（死亡）人数} \times 100$$

3.2.7 累积发病（死亡）率

累积发病（死亡）率是指某病在某一年龄阶段内按年龄（岁）进行累积的发病（死亡）率总指标。累积发病（死亡）率消除了年龄构成不同的影响，故不需要标准化便可以直接用于不同地区的比较。恶性肿瘤一般是计算 0~74 岁的累积发病（死亡）率。

$$累积发病（死亡）率（\%）=（\Sigma[年龄组发病（死亡）率 \times 年龄组距]）\times 100$$

Direct method in calculating age-standardized incidence（mortality）rate:

（1）Calculate the rate for cases in a specific age group in a target population.

（2）Calculate the weighted age-specific rates. The weights applied represent the relative age distribution of the standard population.

（3）Add up each weighted age-specific rate. The sum of rates reflects the adjusted rate.

$$ASR\ per\ 100\,000 = \frac{\Sigma(standard\ population\ in\ corresponding\ age\ group \times age\text{-}specific\ rate)}{\Sigma\ standard\ population} \times 100{,}000$$

3.2.6 Relative frequency

The relative frequency indicates the percentage of the number of site-specific new cancer cases（deaths）accounting in the numbers of all cancers combined. The formula is:

$$Relative\ frequency\ of\ a\ certain\ type\ of\ cancer（\%）= \frac{No.\ of\ cases（deaths）of\ a\ particular\ cancer}{No.\ of\ cases（deaths）of\ all\ cancers} \times 100$$

3.2.7 Cumulative rate

The cumulative rate indicates the probability of the onset of a cancer between birth and a specific age. The cumulative incidence（mortality）rate eliminates the influence of age structure, so it can be directly compared in different regions without standardization. The cumulative rate of cancer is often calculated for population between 0 and 74 years.

$$Cumulative\ rate（\%）=[\Sigma(age\text{-}specific\ rate \times width\ of\ the\ age\ group）]\times 100$$

（撰稿 王宁，校稿 杨雷）

4 2019 年北京市恶性肿瘤发病与死亡
Incidence and Mortality for Cancers in Beijing, 2019

4.1 北京市肿瘤登记覆盖人口

　　2019 年北京市年中户籍人口数为 13 866 241 人（男性 6 894 578 人，女性 6 971 663 人）。其中，城区人口 8 543 242 人（男性 4 241 884 人，女性 4 301 358 人），占全市人口的 61.61%；郊区人口 5 322 999 人（男性 2 652 694 人，女性 2 670 305 人），占全市人口的 38.39%（表 4.1.1，图 4.1.1 至图 4.1.3）。

4.1 Population coverage of BCR

　　In 2019, the number of mid-year population with household registration of Beijing was 13,866,241 (6,894,578 for males and 6,971,663 for females), for urban areas 8,543,242 (4,241,884 for males and 4,301,358 for females), or 61.61% of the total; and for peri-urban areas 5,322,999 (2,652,694 for males and 2,670,305 for females), or 38.39% of the total (Table 4.1.1, Figure 4.1.1-4.1.3).

表 4.1.1 2019 年北京市肿瘤登记覆盖人口
Table 4.1.1 Population in different areas of Beijing in 2019

年龄组 Age group（years）	全市 All areas			城区 Urban areas			郊区 Peri-urban areas		
	男性 Male	女性 Female	合计 Both	男性 Male	女性 Female	合计 Both	男性 Male	女性 Female	合计 Both
合计 Total	6 894 578	6 971 663	13 866 241	4 241 884	4 301 358	8 543 242	2 652 694	2 670 305	5 322 999
0~	68 615	64 087	132 702	35 859	33 397	69 256	32 756	30 690	63 446
1~	336 642	314 987	651 629	196 545	183 055	379 600	140 097	131 932	272 029
5~	346 342	324 100	670 442	216 450	202 036	418 486	129 892	122 064	251 956
10~	241 401	226 337	467 738	146 216	136 488	282 704	95 185	89 849	185 034
15~	209 014	203 462	412 476	129 732	127 208	256 940	79 282	76 254	155 536
20~	304 510	304 597	609 107	197 306	200 796	398 102	107 204	103 801	211 005
25~	399 047	390 483	789 530	241 116	235 771	476 887	157 931	154 712	312 643
30~	581 294	580 677	1 161 971	326 506	327 362	653 868	254 788	253 315	508 103
35~	599 918	597 246	1 197 164	374 239	379 093	753 332	225 679	218 153	443 832

年龄组 Age group （years）	全市 All areas			城区 Urban areas			郊区 Peri-urban areas		
	男性 Male	女性 Female	合计 Both	男性 Male	女性 Female	合计 Both	男性 Male	女性 Female	合计 Both
40～	427 466	416 519	843 985	269 118	263 211	532 329	158 348	153 308	311 656
45～	524 452	524 866	1 049 318	305 413	308 783	614 196	219 039	216 083	435 122
50～	519 527	515 642	1 035 169	295 660	291 444	587 104	223 867	224 198	448 065
55～	619 966	607 997	1 227 963	390 470	375 217	765 687	229 496	232 780	462 276
60～	566 676	588 742	1 155 418	362 217	375 517	737 734	204 459	213 225	417 684
65～	438 201	470 457	908 658	276 579	293 004	569 583	161 622	177 453	339 075
70～	250 013	279 594	529 607	152 177	168 944	321 121	97 836	110 650	208 486
75～	171 849	211 169	383 018	110 589	139 473	250 062	61 260	71 696	132 956
80～	158 720	193 126	351 846	113 420	141 852	255 272	45 300	51 274	96 574
85+	130 925	157 575	288 500	102 272	118 707	220 979	28 653	38 868	67 521

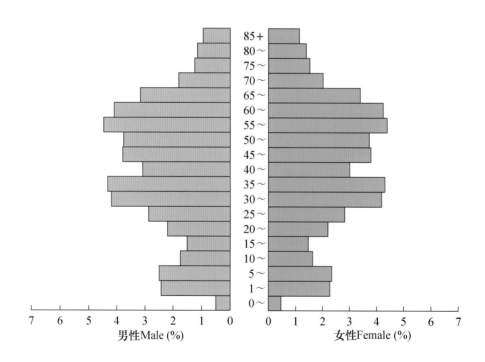

图 4.1.1 2019 年北京市人口金字塔
Figure 4.1.1 Population pyramid in Beijing, 2019

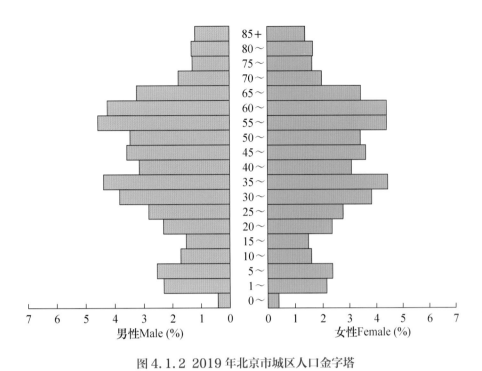

图 4.1.2 2019 年北京市城区人口金字塔
Figure 4.1.2 Population pyramid in urban areas of Beijing, 2019

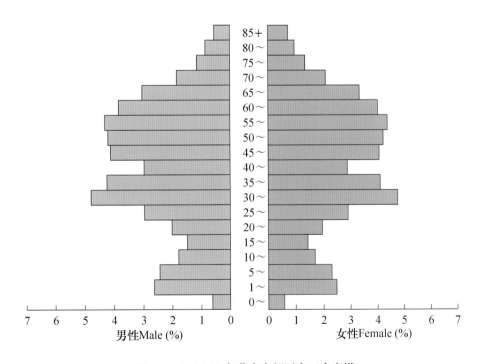

图 4.1.3 2019 年北京市郊区人口金字塔
Figure 4.1.3 Population pyramid in peri-urban areas of Beijing, 2019

4.2 北京市全部恶性肿瘤发病和死亡

4.2.1 北京市全部恶性肿瘤发病情况

2019年北京市新发病例数 58 234 例（男性 28 571 例，女性 29 663 例），其中城区新发病例数为 38 069 例，占 65.37%，郊区 20 165 例，占 34.63%。全市发病率为 419.97/10 万（男性 414.40/10 万，女性 425.48/10 万），中标发病率为 226.25/10 万，世标发病率为 215.95/10 万，0～74 岁累积发病率为 23.76%。城区发病率为 445.60/10 万（男性 436.08/10 万，女性 455.00/10 万），中标率发病率为 232.47/10 万，世标发病率为 221.72/10 万，0～74 岁累积发病率为 24.46%。郊区发病率为 378.83/10 万（男性 379.73/10 万，女性 377.93/10 万），中标率发病率为 216.50/10 万，世标发病率为 206.78/10 万，0～74 岁累积发病率为 22.63%。城区与郊区相比，城区男性和女性发病率、中标发病率、世标发病率以及 0～74 岁累积发病率均高于郊区相应指标（表 4.2.1）。

北京市全部恶性肿瘤世标发病率由 2010 年的 163.31 /10 万上升到 2019 年的 215.95/10 万，年均变化百分比为 2.54%（$P < 0.001$）；男性和女性世标发病率 10 年间年均变化百分比分别为 1.41%（$P = 0.004$）和 3.65%（$P < 0.001$）。

4.2 Incidence and mortality for all cancer sites in Beijing

4.2.1 Incidence of all cancer sites in Beijing

In 2019, there were 58,234 new cases（28,571 for males and 29,663 for females）in Beijing, 38,069（65.37%）in urban areas and 20,165（34.63%）in peri-urban areas. The incidence rate of all cancers was 419.97 per 100,000（414.40 per 100,000 for males and 425.48 per 100,000 for females）, with an ASR China of 226.25 per 100,000, an ASR World of 215.95 per 100,000, and a cumulative rate for subjects aged 0 to 74 years of 23.76%. The incidence rate of all cancers in urban areas was 445.60 per 100,000（436.08 per 100,000 for males and 455.00 per 100,000 for females）, with an ASR China of 232.47 per 100,000, an ASR World of 221.72 per 100,000, and a cumulative rate for subjects aged 0 to 74 years of 24.46%. The incidence rate of all cancers in peri-urban areas was 378.83 per 100,000（379.73 per 100,000 for males and 377.93 per 100,000 for females）, with an ASR China of 216.50 per 100,000, an ASR World of 206.78 per 100,000, and a cumulative rate for subjects aged 0 to 74 years of 22.63%. The crude incidence rates, ASRs China for incidence, ASRs World for incidence and cumulative incidence rates of all cancer sites were all higher in urban areas than those in peri-urban areas for both sexes（Table 4.2.1）.

The ASR World for incidence of all cancers increased from 163.31 per 100,000 in 2010 to 215.95 per 100,000 in 2019; and the annual percentage change（APC）was 2.54%（$P < 0.001$）. The APCs in the last 10 years for males and females were 1.41%（$P = 0.004$）and 3.65%（$P < 0.001$）, respectively.

表 4.2.1 2019 年北京市户籍居民全部恶性肿瘤发病情况
Table 4.2.1 Incidence of all cancer sites in Beijing, 2019

地区 Area	性别 Sex	例数 No. of cases	发病率 Incidence rate （1/10^5）	中标率 ASR China （1/10^5）	世标率 ASR World （1/10^5）	累积率 Cumulative rate （0~74, %）
全市 All areas	合计 Both	58 234	419.97	226.25	215.95	23.76
	男性 Male	28 571	414.40	209.50	204.52	23.47
	女性 Female	29 663	425.48	245.48	229.68	24.25
城区 Urban areas	合计 Both	38 069	445.60	232.47	221.72	24.46
	男性 Male	18 498	436.08	211.52	205.89	23.67
	女性 Female	19 571	455.00	255.66	239.63	25.42
郊区 Peri-urban areas	合计 Both	20 165	378.83	216.50	206.78	22.63
	男性 Male	10 073	379.73	206.47	202.48	23.13
	女性 Female	10 092	377.93	229.54	214.00	22.42

4.2.2 北京市全部恶性肿瘤年龄别发病率

2019 年北京市全部恶性肿瘤的年龄别发病率在 0~19 岁时处于较低水平，自 20~24 岁年龄组开始快速上升，在 80~84 岁年龄组达到高峰。除 0~ 和 1~4 岁组外，60 岁之前女性年龄别发病率始终高于男性，自 60 岁之后男性发病率高于女性。城区和郊区恶性肿瘤年龄别发病率变化趋势基本相同。30 岁以下和 80 岁以上城区和郊区各年龄组发病率差异不明显，30~79 岁各年龄组城区发病率均高于郊区（表 4.2.2，图 4.2.1 至图 4.2.3）。

4.2.2 Age-specific incidence rates of all cancer sites in Beijing

Age-specific incidence rates were relatively low at the age group of 0-19 years, and increased sharply from the age group of 20-24 years, which peaked at the age group of 80-84 years. Except for the age groups of 0- and 1-4 years, age-specific incidence rates were consistently higher in females than those in males before 60 years old, and since then the age-specific incidence rates for males exceeded those for females. The overall trend of age-specific incidence rate in urban areas was similar to that in peri-urban areas. The age-specific incidence rates were similar in urban and peri-urban areas for people below 30 years and above 80 years old, but were higher in urban areas than those in peri-urban areas in people of age groups of 30-79 years (Table 4.2.2, Figure 4.2.1-4.2.3).

表 4.2.2 2019 年北京市户籍居民恶性肿瘤年龄别发病率（1/10⁵）

Table 4.2.2 Age-specific incidence rates of all cancer sites in Beijing, 2019（1/10⁵）

年龄组 Age group （years）	全市 All areas			城区 Urban areas			郊区 Peri-urban areas		
	合计 Both	男性 Male	女性 Female	合计 Both	男性 Male	女性 Female	合计 Both	男性 Male	女性 Female
合计 Total	419.97	414.40	425.48	445.60	436.08	455.00	378.83	379.73	377.93
0~	19.59	23.32	15.60	21.66	22.31	20.96	17.34	24.42	9.78
1~	18.88	19.90	17.78	18.97	18.32	19.67	18.75	22.13	15.16
5~	11.04	10.97	11.11	12.66	11.55	13.86	8.33	10.01	6.55
10~	8.34	6.21	10.60	8.14	6.16	10.26	8.65	6.30	11.13
15~	14.30	11.48	17.20	14.79	10.02	19.65	13.50	13.87	13.11
20~	33.82	22.66	44.98	31.90	21.79	41.83	37.44	24.25	51.06
25~	92.84	63.15	123.18	94.57	63.87	125.97	90.20	62.05	118.93
30~	121.78	82.40	161.19	131.68	92.49	170.76	109.03	69.47	148.83
35~	172.99	109.68	236.59	181.06	117.30	244.00	159.29	97.04	223.70
40~	242.42	137.55	350.04	247.97	141.95	356.37	232.95	130.09	339.19
45~	316.11	195.44	436.68	320.42	191.87	447.56	310.03	200.42	421.13
50~	398.29	305.09	492.20	408.28	295.27	522.91	385.21	318.05	452.28
55~	562.96	531.16	595.40	583.92	532.18	637.76	528.26	529.42	527.11
60~	722.94	783.87	664.30	750.27	799.52	702.76	674.67	756.14	596.55
65~	909.80	1 057.96	771.80	935.77	1 079.26	800.33	866.18	1021.52	724.70
70~	1 124.42	1 356.33	917.04	1 150.66	1 351.06	970.14	1 084.01	1364.53	835.97
75~	1 356.59	1 658.43	1 110.96	1 371.26	1 663.82	1 139.29	1 329.01	1 648.71	1 055.85
80~	1 507.19	1 842.87	1 231.32	1 506.63	1 833.01	1 245.66	1 508.69	1 867.55	1 191.64
85+	1 391.68	1 694.10	1 140.41	1 391.08	1 656.37	1 162.53	1 393.64	1 828.78	1 072.86

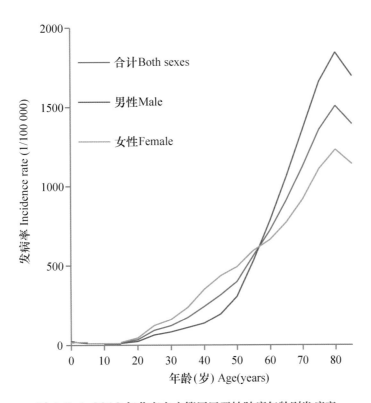

图 4.2.1 2019 年北京市户籍居民恶性肿瘤年龄别发病率
Figure 4.2.1 Age-specific incidence rates of all cancer sites in Beijing, 2019

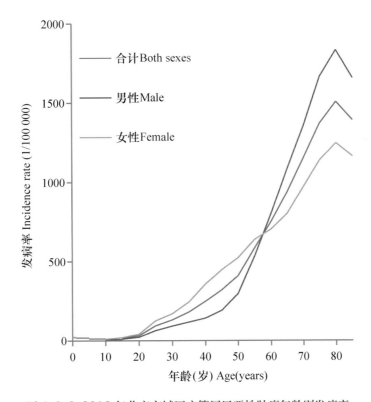

图 4.2.2 2019 年北京市城区户籍居民恶性肿瘤年龄别发病率
Figure 4.2.2 Age-specific incidence rates of all cancer sites in urban areas of Beijing, 2019

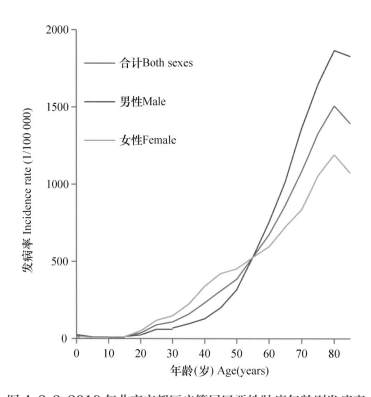

图 4.2.3 2019 年北京市郊区户籍居民恶性肿瘤年龄别发病率
Figure 4.2.3 Age-specific incidence rates of all cancer sites in peri-urban areas of Beijing, 2019

4.2.3 北京市全部恶性肿瘤死亡情况

2019 年，北京市恶性肿瘤死亡报告 27 350 例（男性 16 203 例，女性 11 147 例）。其中，城区 17 848 例，占全市恶性肿瘤死亡的 65.26%，郊区 9 502 例，占全部恶性肿瘤死亡的 34.74%。北京市 2019 年恶性肿瘤死亡率为 197.24/10 万（男性 235.01/10 万，女性 159.89/10 万），中标死亡率为 78.78/10 万，世标死亡率为 78.35/10 万，0~74 岁累积死亡率为 8.20%。城区死亡率为 208.91/10 万（男性 244.40/10 万，女性 173.92/10 万），中标死亡率为 76.04/10 万，世标死亡率为 75.81/10 万，0~74 岁累积死亡率为 7.88%。郊区死亡率为 178.51/10 万（男性 220.00/10 万，女性 137.29/10 万），中标死亡率为 83.25/10 万，世标死亡率为 82.38/10 万，

4.2.3 Mortality of all cancer sites in Beijing

In 2019, there were 27,350 cancer deaths（16,203 for males and 11,147 for females）in Beijing, with 17,848 deaths（65.26%）in urban areas and 9,502 deaths（34.74%）in peri-urban areas. The mortality rate of all cancer sites was 197.24 per 100,000 in 2019（235.01 per 100,000 for males and 159.89 per 100,000 for females）, with an ASR China of 78.78 per 100,000, an ASR World of 78.35 per 100,000, and a cumulative mortality rate for subjects aged 0 to 74 years of 8.20%. The mortality rate of all cancers in urban areas was 208.91 per 100,000（244.40 per 100,000 for males and 173.92 per 100,000 for females）, with an ASR China of 76.04 per 100,000, an ASR World of 75.81 per 100,000, and a cumulative rate for subjects aged 0 to 74 years of 7.88%. The mortality rate of all cancer sites in peri-urban areas was 178.51 per 100,000（220.00 per 100,000 for males and 137.29 per 100,000 for females）, with an ASR China of 83.25 per 100,000, an ASR World of 82.38 per 100,000, and a cumulative rate for subjects aged 0 to 74 years of 8.69%. The crude mortality rates of all cancer

0～74 岁累积死亡率为 8.69%。城区和郊区相比，城区男性和女性死亡率均高于郊区，但城区男性和女性的中标死亡率、世标死亡率和 0～74 岁累积死亡率均低于郊区（表 4.2.3）。

北京市全部恶性肿瘤世标死亡率由 2010 年的 89.84 /10 万下降到 2019 年的 78.35 /10 万，年均变化百分比为 -1.42%（$P < 0.001$）；男性和女性世标死亡率 10 年间年均变化百分比分别为 -1.13%（$P = 0.002$）和 -1.75%（$P < 0.001$）。

sites were higher in the urban areas than those in the peri-urban areas for both sexes. However, the ASR China and ASR World for mortality and cumulative mortality rate were lower in urban areas than those in peri-urban areas (Table 4.2.3).

The ASR World for mortality of all cancers decreased from 89.84 per 100,000 in 2010 to 78.35 per 100,000 in 2019, with an APC of -1.42%（$P < 0.001$）during the period of time. And the APCs in the last 10 years for males and females were -1.13%（$P = 0.002$）and -1.75%（$P < 0.001$）, respectively.

表 4.2.3 2019 年北京市户籍居民全部恶性肿瘤死亡情况
Table 4.2.3 Mortality of all cancer sites in Beijing, 2019

地区 Area	性别 Sex	例数 No. of deaths	死亡率 Mortality rate （1/10^5）	中标率 ASR China （1/10^5）	世标率 ASR World （1/10^5）	累积率 Cumulative rate （0～74,%）
全市 All areas	合计 Both	27 350	197.24	78.78	78.35	8.20
	男性 Male	16 203	235.01	98.25	98.31	10.57
	女性 Female	11 147	159.89	61.23	60.23	5.98
城区 Urban areas	合计 Both	17 848	208.91	76.04	75.81	7.88
	男性 Male	10 367	244.40	93.03	93.43	9.97
	女性 Female	7 481	173.92	60.76	59.77	5.91
郊区 Peri-urban areas	合计 Both	9 502	178.51	83.25	82.38	8.69
	男性 Male	5 836	220.00	106.97	106.46	11.50
	女性 Female	3 666	137.29	61.85	60.71	6.11

4.2.4 北京市全部恶性肿瘤年龄别死亡率

北京市恶性肿瘤年龄别死亡率在 40 岁以前处于较低水平，自 40～44 岁年龄组开始年龄别死亡率快速上升，在 85 岁及以上年龄组达到高峰。自 45～49 岁年龄组开始，男性年龄别死亡率始终高于女性。城区和郊区年龄别死亡率的变化趋势基本相同。45 岁以下城区和郊区各年龄组死亡率差异不明显，45 岁以上各年龄组除 85 岁及以上年龄组外，郊区各年龄组死亡率均高于城区（表 4.2.4，图 4.2.4 至图 4.2.6）。

4.2.4 Age-specific mortality rates of all cancer sites in Beijing

Age-specific mortality rates were relatively low before 40 years old, and increased dramatically since then, which peaked at the age group of 85 years and above. Age-specific mortality rates were consistently higher in males than those in females since the age group of 45-49 years. The overall trend of age-specific mortality rate in urban areas was similar to that in peri-urban areas. The age-specific mortality rates were similar in urban and peri-urban areas in people below 45 years old, but higher in peri-urban areas above 45 years old, except for the age group of 85 years and above（Table 4.2.4, Figure 4.2.4-4.2.6）.

表 4.2.4 2019 年北京市户籍居民恶性肿瘤年龄别死亡率（$1/10^5$）
Table 4.2.4 Age-specific mortality rates of all cancer sites in Beijing, 2019（$1/10^5$）

年龄组 Age group （years）	全市 All areas			城区 Urban areas			郊区 Peri-urban areas		
	合计 Both	男性 Male	女性 Female	合计 Both	男性 Male	女性 Female	合计 Both	男性 Male	女性 Female
合计 Total	197.24	235.01	159.89	208.91	244.40	173.92	178.51	220.00	137.29
0～	3.01	5.83	0.00	4.33	8.37	0.00	1.58	3.05	0.00
1～	2.00	2.97	0.95	2.37	3.05	1.64	1.47	2.86	0.00
5～	2.24	2.31	2.16	1.67	1.85	1.48	3.18	3.08	3.28
10～	1.50	1.66	1.33	1.06	0.68	1.47	2.16	3.15	1.11
15～	2.91	3.35	2.46	1.17	2.31	0.00	5.79	5.05	6.56
20～	3.45	2.63	4.27	3.77	3.04	4.48	2.84	1.87	3.85
25～	5.19	5.51	4.87	4.61	4.15	5.09	6.08	7.60	4.52
30～	9.38	9.12	9.64	9.33	8.88	9.78	9.45	9.42	9.47
35～	15.95	13.84	18.08	16.33	12.56	20.05	15.32	15.95	14.67
40～	26.66	23.63	29.77	27.24	24.15	30.39	25.67	22.73	28.70

续表

年龄组 Age group （years）	全市 All areas			城区 Urban areas			郊区 Peri-urban areas		
	合计 Both	男性 Male	女性 Female	合计 Both	男性 Male	女性 Female	合计 Both	男性 Male	女性 Female
45~	53.75	55.11	52.39	48.36	45.51	51.17	61.36	68.48	54.15
50~	95.25	113.76	76.60	89.59	101.13	77.89	102.66	130.43	74.93
55~	167.43	207.43	126.65	163.38	197.71	127.66	174.14	223.97	125.01
60~	265.27	359.11	174.95	256.60	350.07	166.44	280.59	375.14	189.94
65~	390.03	519.85	269.10	381.68	505.82	264.50	404.04	543.86	276.69
70~	598.18	793.16	423.83	568.32	732.70	420.26	644.17	887.20	429.28
75~	930.24	1 178.94	727.85	888.58	1 115.84	708.38	1 008.60	1 292.85	765.73
80~	1 395.21	1 719.38	1 128.80	1 367.56	1 659.32	1 134.28	1 468.30	1 869.76	1 113.62
85+	1 683.54	2 051.56	1 377.76	1 709.66	2 038.68	1 426.20	1 598.02	2 097.51	1 229.80

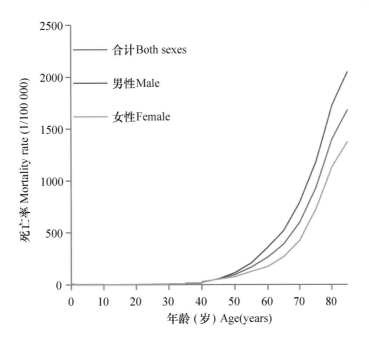

图 4.2.4 2019 年北京市户籍居民恶性肿瘤年龄别死亡率

Figure 4.2.4 Age-specific mortality rates of all cancer sites in Beijing, 2019

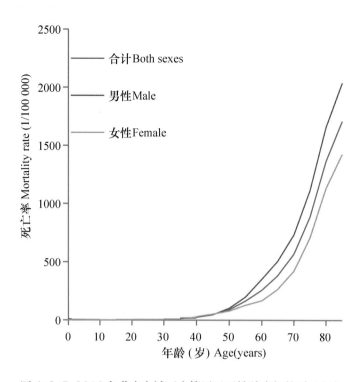

图 4.2.5 2019 年北京市城区户籍居民恶性肿瘤年龄别死亡率
Figure 4.2.5 Age-specific mortality rates of all cancer sites in urban areas of Beijing, 2019

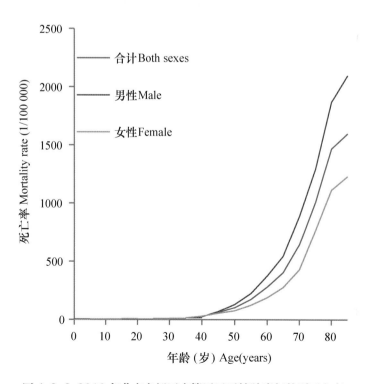

图 4.2.6 2019 年北京市郊区户籍居民恶性肿瘤年龄别死亡率
Figure 4.2.6 Age-specific mortality rates of all cancer sites in peri-urban areas of Beijing, 2019

4.2.5 北京市全部恶性肿瘤地区分布

2019年，北京市16个辖区恶性肿瘤世标发病率和死亡率呈现明显的差异，城区世标发病率高于郊区，郊区世标死亡率高于城区（图4.2.7和图4.2.8）。

4.2.5 Incidence and mortality rates of all cancer sites by district of Beijing

In 2019, there were significant differences among the 16 districts in ASR World for incidence and mortality of all cancers in Beijing. The incidence rate was higher in urban areas than that in peri-urban areas, while the mortality rate was higher in peri-urban areas than that in urban areas（Figure 4.2.7-4.2.8）.

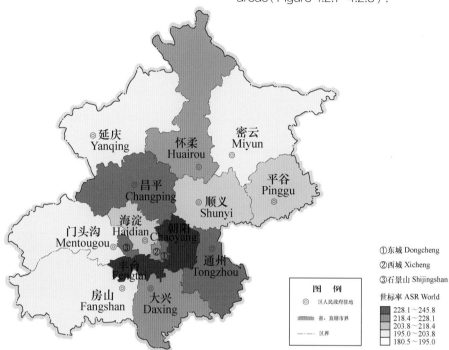

图 4.2.7 2019 年北京市户籍居民全部恶性肿瘤世标发病率（1/10^5）地区分布情况
Figure 4.2.7 ASRs World for incidence of all cancer sites（1/10^5）by district in Beijing, 2019

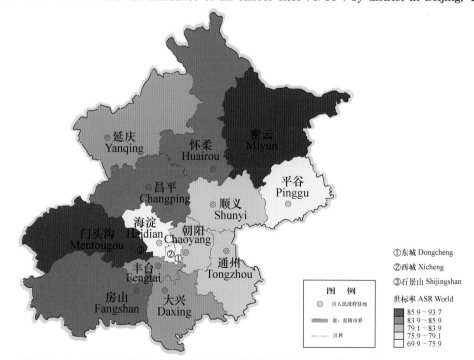

图 4.2.8 2019 年北京市户籍居民全部恶性肿瘤世标死亡率（1/10^5）地区分布情况
Figure 4.2.8 ASRs World for mortality rates of all cancer sites（1/10^5）by district in Beijing, 2019

4.3 北京市前 10 位恶性肿瘤发病与死亡

4.3.1 北京市前 10 位恶性肿瘤发病情况

2019 年，北京市男性恶性肿瘤发病第 1 位的是肺癌，后依次为结直肠癌、胃癌、甲状腺癌和前列腺癌。女性恶性肿瘤发病第 1 位的是乳腺癌，后依次为肺癌、甲状腺癌、结直肠癌和子宫体癌（表 4.3.1，图 4.3.1 至图 4.3.4）。

4.3 Top 10 cancer sites in terms of incidence and mortality in Beijing

4.3.1 Top 10 cancer sites in terms of incidence in Beijing

In 2019, the most common cancer for males was lung cancer, followed by colorectal, stomach, thyroid and prostate cancers. The most common cancer for females was breast cancer, followed by lung, thyroid, colorectal, and uterus cancers（Table 4.3.1, Figure 4.3.1-4.3.4）.

表 4.3.1　2019 年北京市户籍居民恶性肿瘤发病前 10 位

Table 4.3.1 Top 10 cancer sites in Beijing in terms of incidence, 2019

顺位 Rank	部位 Site	例数 No. of cases	构成比 Freq.（%）	粗率 Crude rate （1/10^5）	中标率 ASR China （1/10^5）	世标率 ASR World （1/10^5）
			男性 Male			
1	肺 Lung	7 148	25.02	103.68	47.00	47.01
2	结直肠 Colon-rectum	4 348	15.22	63.06	29.35	29.25
3	胃 Stomach	1 820	6.37	26.40	11.82	11.75
4	甲状腺 Thyroid	1 799	6.30	26.09	25.10	20.30
5	前列腺 Prostate	1 798	6.29	26.08	11.04	10.86
6	肝 Liver	1 750	6.13	25.38	12.38	12.41
7	肾 Kidney	1 504	5.26	21.81	11.71	11.55
8	膀胱 Bladder	1 473	5.16	21.36	9.45	9.42
9	食管 Esophagus	933	3.27	13.53	5.97	6.11
10	淋巴瘤 Lymphoma	919	3.22	13.33	7.04	6.80

女性 Female					
部位 Site	例数 No. of cases	构成比 Freq. （%）	粗率 Crude rate （1/10^5）	中标率 ASR China （1/10^5）	世标率 ASR World （1/10^5）
乳腺 Breast	5 949	20.06	85.33	52.17	48.92
肺 Lung	5 498	18.53	78.86	36.38	35.64
甲状腺 Thyroid	4 445	14.98	63.76	58.73	49.27
结直肠 Colon-rectum	3 001	10.12	43.05	19.02	18.56
子宫体 Uterus	1 523	5.13	21.85	12.79	12.38
肾 Kidney	875	2.95	12.55	5.91	5.72
卵巢 Ovary	851	2.87	12.21	7.59	7.26
胃 Stomach	815	2.75	11.69	5.21	5.00
胰腺 Pancreas	773	2.61	11.09	4.28	4.24
淋巴瘤 Lymphoma	743	2.50	10.66	5.61	5.38

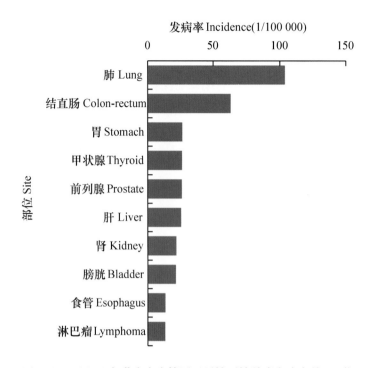

图 4.3.1　2019 年北京市户籍居民男性恶性肿瘤发病率前 10 位
Figure 4.3.1 Top 10 cancer sites in terms of incidence for males in Beijing, 2019

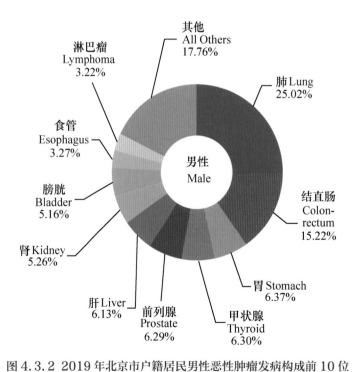

图 4.3.2　2019 年北京市户籍居民男性恶性肿瘤发病构成前 10 位
Figure 4.3.2 Distribution of the top 10 cancer sites in terms of incidence for males in Beijing, 2019

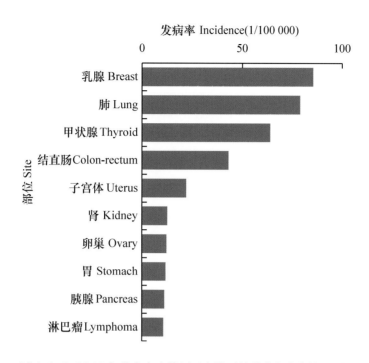

图 4.3.3 2019 年北京市户籍居民女性恶性肿瘤发病率前 10 位
Figure 4.3.3 Top 10 cancer sites in terms of incidence for females in Beijing, 2019

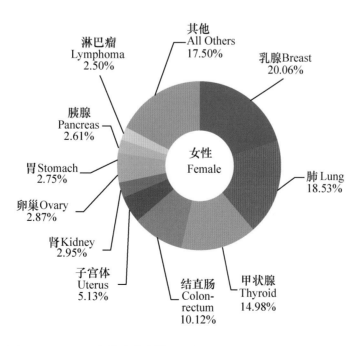

图 4.3.4 2019 年北京市户籍居民女性恶性肿瘤发病构成前 10 位
Figure 4.3.4 Distribution of the top 10 cancer sites in terms of incidence for females in Beijing, 2019

4.3.2 北京市前 10 位恶性肿瘤死亡情况

2019 年，北京市男性和女性恶性肿瘤死亡第 1 位的均为肺癌，其次为结直肠癌。男性恶性肿瘤死亡第 3~5 位的分别为肝癌、胃癌和食管癌，女性分别为乳腺癌、胰腺癌和胃癌（表 4.3.2，图 4.3.5 至图 4.3.8）。

4.3.2 Top 10 cancer sites in terms of mortality in Beijing

For both sexes, lung cancer was the leading cause of cancer deaths, followed by colorectal cancer. As for males, liver cancer, stomach cancer, and esophagus cancer were the 3rd, 4th, and 5th leading causes of deaths in all cancers, respectively. And for females, breast cancer, pancreas cancer, and stomach cancer were the 3rd, 4th, and 5th leading causes of cancer deaths, respectively (Table 4.3.2, Figure 4.3.5-4.3.8) .

表 4.3.2　2019 年北京市户籍居民恶性肿瘤死亡前 10 位

Table 4.3.2　Top 10 cancer sites in terms of mortality in Beijing, 2019

顺位 Rank	部位 Site	例数 No. of deaths	构成比 Freq. (%)	粗率 Crude rate (1/10^5)	中标率 ASR China (1/10^5)	世标率 ASR World (1/10^5)
			男性 Male			
1	肺 Lung	5 112	31.55	74.15	30.78	30.64
2	结直肠 Colon-rectum	1 812	11.18	26.28	10.50	10.41
3	肝 Liver	1 424	8.79	20.65	9.62	9.60
4	胃 Stomach	1 307	8.07	18.96	7.64	7.64
5	食管 Esophagus	805	4.97	11.68	4.91	5.02
6	胰腺 Pancreas	739	4.56	10.72	4.67	4.69
7	前列腺 Prostate	694	4.28	10.07	3.12	3.20
8	淋巴瘤 Lymphoma	599	3.70	8.69	4.17	4.11
9	白血病 Leukemia	589	3.64	8.54	3.64	3.61
10	膀胱 Bladder	570	3.52	8.27	2.73	2.81

女性 Female					
部位 Site	例数 No. of deaths	构成比 Freq.（%）	粗率 Crude rate （1/10^5）	中标率 ASR China （1/10^5）	世标率 ASR World （1/10^5）
肺 Lung	2 698	24.20	38.70	13.35	13.09
结直肠 Colon-rectum	1 350	12.11	19.36	6.61	6.56
乳腺 Breast	1 167	10.47	16.74	7.38	7.23
胰腺 Pancreas	706	6.33	10.13	3.65	3.61
胃 Stomach	600	5.38	8.61	3.39	3.26
肝 Liver	542	4.86	7.77	2.75	2.75
胆囊 Gallbladder	499	4.48	7.16	2.49	2.46
卵巢 Ovary	486	4.36	6.97	3.28	3.27
淋巴瘤 Lymphoma	431	3.87	6.18	2.45	2.41
白血病 Leukemia	358	3.21	5.14	2.36	2.28

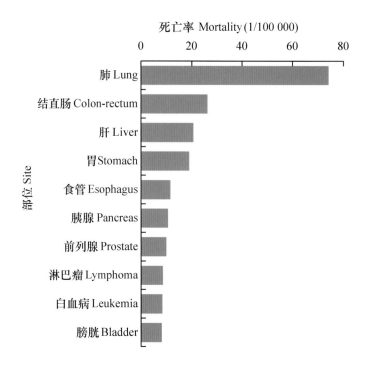

图 4.3.5 2019 年北京市户籍居民男性恶性肿瘤死亡率前 10 位
Figure 4.3.5 Top 10 cancer sites in terms of mortality for males in Beijing, 2019

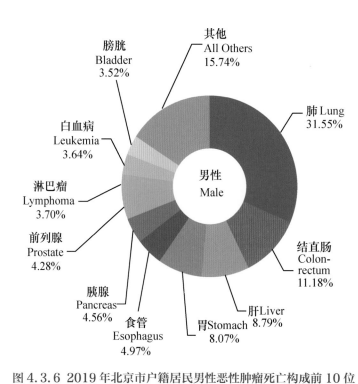

图 4.3.6 2019 年北京市户籍居民男性恶性肿瘤死亡构成前 10 位
Figure 4.3.6 Distribution of the top 10 cancer sites in terms of mortality for males in Beijing, 2019

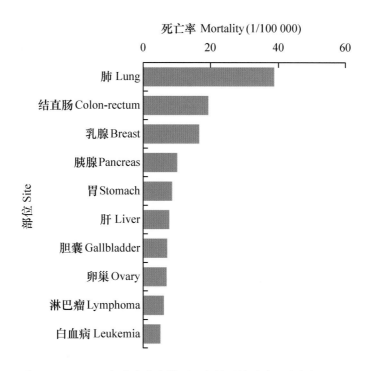

图 4.3.7 2019 年北京市户籍居民女性恶性肿瘤死亡率前 10 位
Figure 4.3.7 Top 10 cancer sites in terms of mortality for females in Beijing, 2019

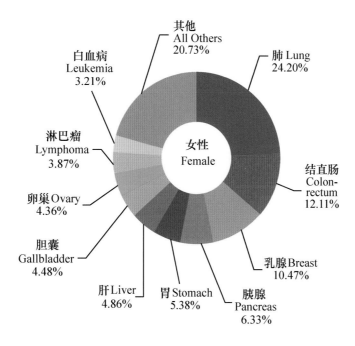

图 4.3.8 2019 年北京市户籍居民女性恶性肿瘤死亡构成前 10 位
Figure 4.3.8 Distribution of the top 10 cancer sites in terms of mortality for females in Beijing, 2019

4.3.3 北京市城区前 10 位恶性肿瘤发病情况

2019 年北京市城区男性恶性肿瘤发病第 1 位的是肺癌，后依次为结直肠癌、前列腺癌、胃癌和甲状腺癌。城区女性恶性肿瘤发病第 1 位的是乳腺癌，后依次为肺癌、甲状腺癌、结直肠癌和子宫体癌（表 4.3.3，图 4.3.9 至图 4.3.12 ）。

4.3.3 Top 10 cancer sites in terms of incidence in urban areas of Beijing

The most common cancer for males was lung cancer in urban areas of Beijing in 2019, followed by colorectal cancer, prostate cancer, stomach cancer, and thyroid cancer. And the most common cancer for females was breast cancer, followed by lung cancer, thyroid cancer, colorectal cancer, and uterus cancer (Table 4.3.3, Figure 4.3.9-4.3.12) .

表 4.3.3 2019 年北京市城区户籍居民恶性肿瘤发病前 10 位
Table 4.3.3 Top 10 cancer sites in terms of incidence in urban areas of Beijing, 2019

顺位 Rank	部位 Site	例数 No. of cases	构成比 Freq.（%）	粗率 Crude rate （1/10^5）	中标率 ASR China （1/10^5）	世标率 ASR World （1/10^5）
			男性 Male			
1	肺 Lung	4 403	23.80	103.80	45.01	45.03
2	结直肠 Colon-rectum	2 939	15.89	69.29	30.72	30.56
3	前列腺 Prostate	1 337	7.23	31.52	12.65	12.45
4	胃 Stomach	1 220	6.60	28.76	12.08	12.03
5	甲状腺 Thyroid	1 191	6.44	28.08	27.49	22.15
6	肝 Liver	1 042	5.63	24.56	11.18	11.26
7	肾 Kidney	1 017	5.50	23.98	12.43	12.11
8	膀胱 Bladder	970	5.24	22.87	9.49	9.45
9	淋巴瘤 Lymphoma	616	3.33	14.52	7.48	7.20
10	胰腺 Pancreas	545	2.95	12.85	5.48	5.51

女性 Female					
部位 Site	例数 No. of cases	构成比 Freq.（%）	粗率 Crude rate （1/10^5）	中标率 ASR China （1/10^5）	世标率 ASR World （1/10^5）
乳腺 Breast	4 098	20.94	95.27	56.32	53.18
肺 Lung	3 579	18.29	83.21	37.79	36.90
甲状腺 Thyroid	2 756	14.08	64.07	60.09	50.19
结直肠 Colon-rectum	2 026	10.35	47.10	19.56	19.14
子宫体 Uterus	977	4.99	22.71	13.14	12.73
肾 Kidney	611	3.12	14.20	6.37	6.16
胃 Stomach	588	3.00	13.67	5.85	5.60
卵巢 Ovary	559	2.86	13.00	8.16	7.79
胰腺 Pancreas	548	2.80	12.74	4.58	4.52
淋巴瘤 Lymphoma	505	2.58	11.74	5.99	5.81

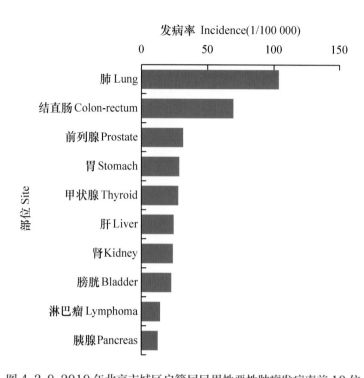

图 4.3.9 2019 年北京市城区户籍居民男性恶性肿瘤发病率前 10 位
Figure 4.3.9 Top 10 cancer sites in terms of incidence for males in urban areas of Beijing, 2019

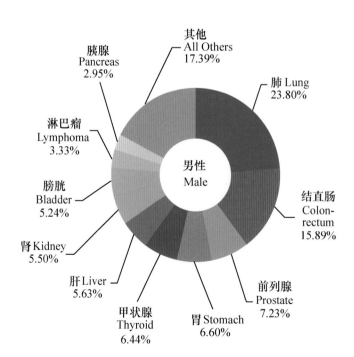

图 4.3.10 2019 年北京市城区户籍居民男性恶性肿瘤发病构成前 10 位
Figure 4.3.10 Distribution of the top 10 cancer sites in terms of incidence for males in urban areas of Beijing, 2019

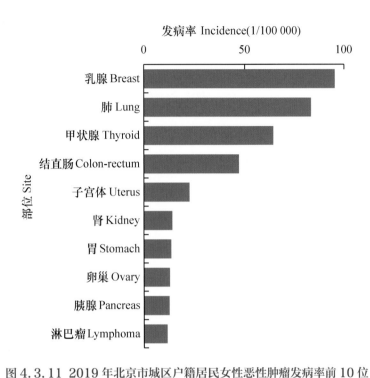

图 4.3.11 2019 年北京市城区户籍居民女性恶性肿瘤发病率前 10 位
Figure 4.3.11 Top 10 cancer sites in terms of incidence for females in urban areas of Beijing, 2019

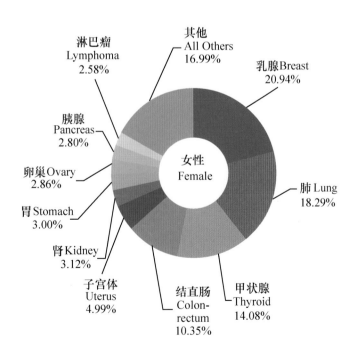

图 4.3.12 2019 年北京市城区户籍居民女性恶性肿瘤发病构成前 10 位
Figure 4.3.12 Distribution of the top 10 cancer sites in terms of incidence for females in urban areas of Beijing, 2019

4.3.4 北京市城区前 10 位恶性肿瘤死亡情况

2019 年，北京市城区男性和女性，恶性肿瘤死亡第 1 位的均为肺癌，其次为结直肠癌。男性恶性肿瘤死亡第 3~5 位的分别为胃癌、肝癌和前列腺癌，女性分别为乳腺癌、胰腺癌和胃癌（表 4.3.4，图 4.3.13 至图 4.3.16）。

4.3.4 Top 10 cancer sites in terms of mortality in urban areas of Beijing

For both sexes, lung cancer was the leading cause of cancer deaths in urban areas of Beijing in 2019, followed by colorectal cancer. Stomach cancer, liver cancer, and prostate cancer were the 3rd, 4th, and 5th leading causes of cancer deaths in all cancers for males, respectively. And for females, breast cancer, pancreas cancer and stomach cancer were the 3rd, 4th, and 5th leading causes of cancer deaths in all cancers, respectively (Table 4.3.4, Figure 4.3.13-4.3.16) .

表 4.3.4 2019 年北京市城区户籍居民恶性肿瘤死亡前 10 位
Table 4.3.4 Top 10 cancer sites in terms of mortality in urban areas of Beijing, 2019

顺位 Rank	部位 Site	男性 Male				
		例数 No. of deaths	构成比 Freq.（%）	粗率 Crude rate （1/10^5）	中标率 ASR China （1/10^5）	世标率 ASR World （1/10^5）
1	肺 Lung	3 088	29.79	72.80	27.86	27.79
2	结直肠 Colon-rectum	1 243	11.99	29.30	10.71	10.67
3	胃 Stomach	874	8.43	20.60	7.49	7.52
4	肝 Liver	840	8.10	19.80	8.49	8.51
5	前列腺 Prostate	517	4.99	12.19	3.25	3.31
6	胰腺 Pancreas	502	4.84	11.83	4.83	4.89
7	食管 Esophagus	439	4.23	10.35	3.94	4.10
8	白血病 Leukemia	417	4.02	9.83	4.28	4.27
9	淋巴瘤 Lymphoma	402	3.88	9.48	3.56	3.52
10	膀胱 Bladder	385	3.71	9.08	2.63	2.72

女性 Female					
部位 Site	例数 No. of deaths	构成比 Freq.（%）	粗率 Crude rate （1/10^5）	中标率 ASR China （1/10^5）	世标率 ASR World （1/10^5）
肺 Lung	1 677	22.42	38.99	11.79	11.54
结直肠 Colon-rectum	975	13.03	22.67	6.95	6.91
乳腺 Breast	864	11.55	20.09	8.08	7.97
胰腺 Pancreas	512	6.84	11.90	3.95	3.91
胃 Stomach	421	5.63	9.79	3.51	3.39
肝 Liver	325	4.34	7.56	2.38	2.40
卵巢 Ovary	324	4.33	7.53	3.37	3.37
淋巴瘤 Lymphoma	302	4.04	7.02	2.68	2.59
胆囊 Gallbladder	301	4.02	7.00	2.18	2.15
肾 Kidney	229	3.06	5.32	1.46	1.47

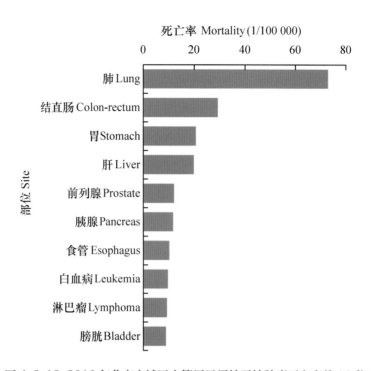

图 4.3.13 2019 年北京市城区户籍居民男性恶性肿瘤死亡率前 10 位

Figure 4.3.13 Top 10 cancer sites in terms of mortality for males in urban areas of Beijing, 2019

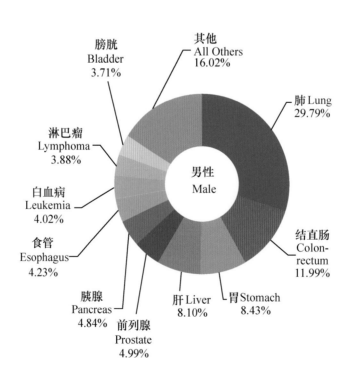

图 4.3.14 2019 年北京市城区户籍居民男性恶性肿瘤死亡构成前 10 位

Figure 4.3.14 Distribution of the top 10 cancer sites in terms of mortality for males in urban areas of Beijing, 2019

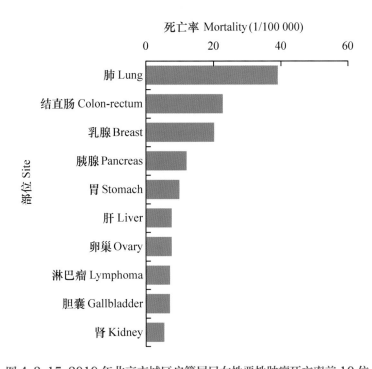

图 4.3.15 2019 年北京市城区户籍居民女性恶性肿瘤死亡率前 10 位
Figure 4.3.15 Top 10 cancer sites in terms of mortality for females in urban areas of Beijing, 2019

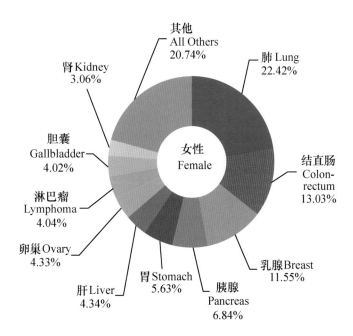

图 4.3.16 2019 年北京市城区户籍居民女性恶性肿瘤死亡构成前 10 位
Figure 4.3.16 Distribution of the top 10 cancer sites in terms of mortality for females in urban areas of Beijing, 2019

4.3.5 北京市郊区前10位恶性肿瘤发病情况

2019年，北京市郊区男性和女性恶性肿瘤发病第1位的均为肺癌。男性恶性肿瘤发病第2~5位的分别为结直肠癌、肝癌、甲状腺癌和胃癌，女性分别为乳腺癌、甲状腺癌、结直肠癌和子宫体癌（表4.3.5，图4.3.17至图4.3.20）。

4.3.5 Top 10 cancer sites in terms of incidence in peri-urban areas of Beijing

For both sexes, lung cancer was the most common cancer in peri-urban area. As for males, colorectal cancer, liver cancer, thyroid cancer and stomach cancer were the 2nd, 3rd, 4th, and 5th most common cancer, respectively. And for females, breast cancer, thyroid cancer, colorectal cancer and uterus cancer were the 2nd, 3rd, 4th, and 5th most common cancer, respectively（Table 4.3.5, Figure 4.3.17-4.3.20）.

表 4.3.5 2019 年北京市郊区户籍居民恶性肿瘤发病前 10 位
Table 4.3.5 Top 10 cancer sites in terms of incidence in peri-urban areas of Beijing, 2019

顺位 Rank	部位 Site	男性 Male				
		例数 No. of cases	构成比 Freq.（%）	粗率 Crude rate （1/10^5）	中标率 ASR China （1/10^5）	世标率 ASR World （1/10^5）
1	肺 Lung	2 745	27.25	103.48	50.71	50.76
2	结直肠 Colon-rectum	1 409	13.99	53.12	27.00	27.03
3	肝 Liver	708	7.03	26.69	14.22	14.17
4	甲状腺 Thyroid	608	6.04	22.92	21.46	17.43
5	胃 Stomach	600	5.96	22.62	11.33	11.23
6	膀胱 Bladder	503	4.99	18.96	9.36	9.37
7	肾 Kidney	487	4.83	18.36	10.48	10.50
8	前列腺 Prostate	461	4.58	17.38	8.20	8.04
9	食管 Esophagus	420	4.17	15.83	7.73	7.73
10	淋巴瘤 Lymphoma	303	3.01	11.42	6.29	6.13

女性 Female					
部位 Site	例数 No. of cases	构成比 Freq.（%）	粗率 Crude rate （1/10^5）	中标率 ASR China （1/10^5）	世标率 ASR World （1/10^5）
肺 Lung	1 919	19.02	71.86	34.50	33.98
乳腺 Breast	1 851	18.34	69.32	45.33	41.89
甲状腺 Thyroid	1 689	16.74	63.25	56.68	47.86
结直肠 Colon-rectum	975	9.66	36.51	17.98	17.46
子宫体 Uterus	546	5.41	20.45	12.29	11.88
卵巢 Ovary	292	2.89	10.94	6.71	6.44
肾 Kidney	264	2.62	9.89	5.11	4.95
肝 Liver	257	2.55	9.62	4.31	4.37
子宫颈 Cervix	257	2.55	9.62	6.89	6.01
淋巴瘤 Lymphoma	238	2.36	8.91	5.02	4.71

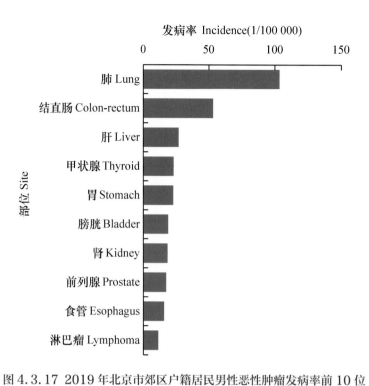

图 4.3.17 2019 年北京市郊区户籍居民男性恶性肿瘤发病率前 10 位
Figure 4.3.17 Top 10 cancer sites in terms of incidence for males in peri-urban areas of Beijing, 2019

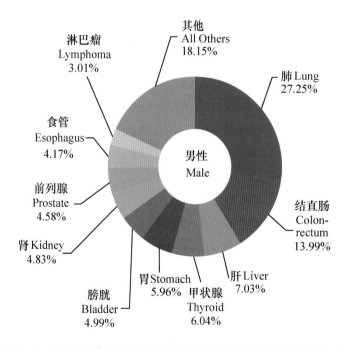

图 4.3.18 2019 年北京市郊区户籍居民男性恶性肿瘤发病构成前 10 位
Figure 4.3.18 Distribution of the top 10 cancer sites in terms of incidence for males in peri-urban areas of Beijing, 2019

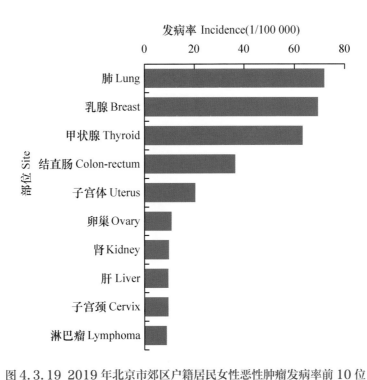

图 4.3.19 2019 年北京市郊区户籍居民女性恶性肿瘤发病率前 10 位
Figure 4.3.19 Top 10 cancer sites in terms of incidence for females in peri-urban areas of Beijing, 2019

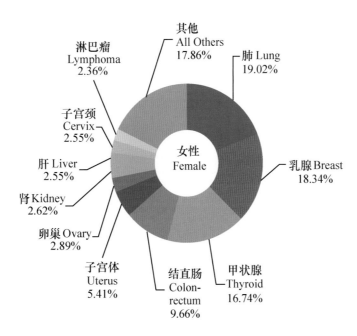

图 4.3.20 2019 年北京市郊区户籍居民女性恶性肿瘤发病构成前 10 位
Figure 4.3.20 Distribution of the top 10 cancer sites in terms of incidence for females in peri-urban areas of Beijing, 2019

4.3.6 北京市郊区前10位恶性肿瘤死亡情况

2019年，北京市郊区男性和女性恶性肿瘤死亡第1位的均为肺癌。男性恶性肿瘤死亡第2～5位的分别为肝癌、结直肠癌、胃癌和食管癌，女性分别为结直肠癌、乳腺癌、肝癌和胆囊癌（表4.3.6，图4.3.21至图4.3.24）。

4.3.6 Top 10 cancer sites in terms of mortality in peri-urban areas of Beijing

For both sexes, lung cancer was the leading cause of cancer deaths in peri-urban areas of Beijing in 2019. As for males, liver cancer, colorectal cancer, stomach cancer, and esophagus cancer were the 2nd, 3rd, 4th, and 5th leading causes of cancer deaths in all cancers, respectively. And for females, colorectal cancer, breast cancer, liver cancer and gallbladder cancer were the 2nd, 3rd, 4th, and 5th leading causes of cancer deaths in all cancers, respectively (Table 4.3.6, Figure 4.3.21- 4.3.24) .

表 4.3.6 2019 年北京市郊区户籍居民恶性肿瘤死亡前 10 位
Table 4.3.6 Top 10 cancer sites in terms of mortality in peri-urban areas of Beijing, 2019

顺位 Rank	部位 Site	例数 No. of deaths	构成比 Freq.（%）	粗率 Crude rate （1/10⁵）	中标率 ASR China （1/10⁵）	世标率 ASR World （1/10⁵）
	男性 Male					
1	肺 Lung	2 024	34.68	76.30	36.06	35.84
2	肝 Liver	584	10.01	22.02	11.35	11.28
3	结直肠 Colon-rectum	569	9.75	21.45	10.21	9.99
4	胃 Stomach	433	7.42	16.32	7.79	7.72
5	食管 Esophagus	366	6.27	13.80	6.60	6.58
6	胰腺 Pancreas	237	4.06	8.93	4.42	4.34
7	胆囊 Gallbladder	221	3.79	8.33	3.92	3.96
8	淋巴瘤 Lymphoma	187	3.20	7.05	3.65	3.62
9	膀胱 Bladder	185	3.17	6.97	2.96	2.99
10	白血病 Leukemia	182	3.12	6.86	3.89	3.80

女性 Female					
部位 Site	例数 No. of deaths	构成比 Freq.（%）	粗率 Crude rate （1/10^5）	中标率 ASR China （1/10^5）	世标率 ASR World （1/10^5）
肺 Lung	1 021	27.85	38.24	16.02	15.73
结直肠 Colon-rectum	375	10.23	14.04	5.94	5.88
乳腺 Breast	303	8.27	11.35	6.02	5.79
肝 Liver	217	5.92	8.13	3.40	3.37
胆囊 Gallbladder	198	5.40	7.41	3.04	3.02
胰腺 Pancreas	194	5.29	7.27	3.09	3.05
胃 Stomach	179	4.88	6.70	3.17	3.00
卵巢 Ovary	162	4.42	6.07	3.12	3.09
淋巴瘤 Lymphoma	129	3.52	4.83	2.06	2.11
白血病 Leukemia	129	3.52	4.83	2.68	2.57

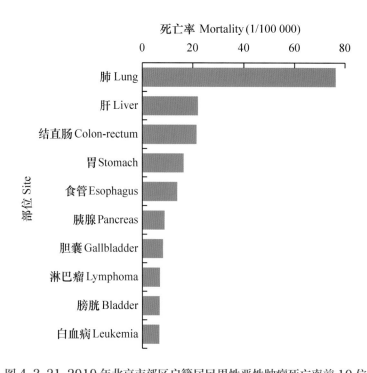

图 4.3.21 2019 年北京市郊区户籍居民男性恶性肿瘤死亡率前 10 位
Figure 4.3.21 Top 10 cancer sites in terms of mortality for males in peri-urban areas of Beijing, 2019

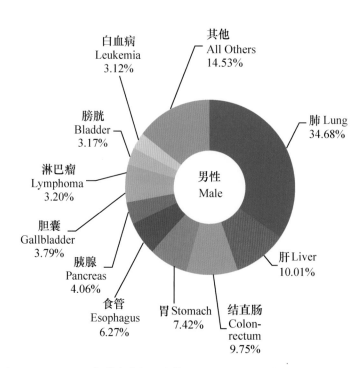

图 4.3.22 2019 年北京市郊区户籍居民男性恶性肿瘤死亡构成前 10 位
Figure 4.3.22 Distribution of the top 10 cancer sites in terms of mortality for males in peri-urban areas of Beijing, 2019

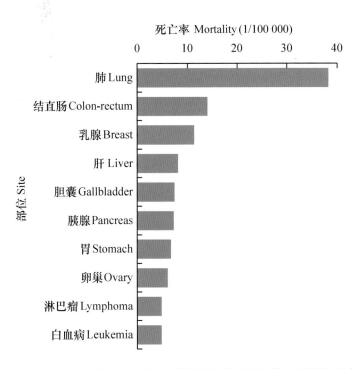

图 4.3.23 2019 年北京市郊区户籍居民女性恶性肿瘤死亡率前 10 位
Figure 4.3.23 Top 10 cancer sites in terms of mortality for females in peri-urban areas of Beijing, 2019

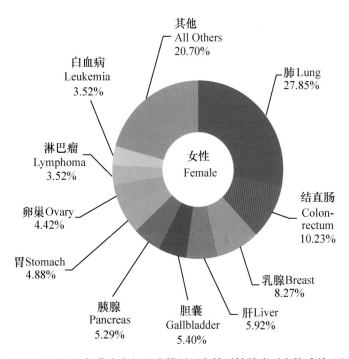

图 4.3.24 2019 年北京市郊区户籍居民女性恶性肿瘤死亡构成前 10 位
Figure 4.3.24 Distribution of the top 10 cancer sites in terms of mortality for females in peri-urban areas of Beijing, 2019

（撰稿 刘硕，校稿 李慧超）

5 各部位恶性肿瘤的发病和死亡
Cancer Incidence and Mortalities by Site

5.1 口腔和咽（C00-10, C12-14）

2019 年，北京市口腔癌和咽癌新发病例数为 769 例，占全部恶性肿瘤发病的 1.32%，位居恶性肿瘤发病第 18 位；其中男性 493 例，女性 276 例，城区 531 例，郊区 238 例。口腔癌和咽癌发病率为 5.55/10 万，中标发病率为 2.84/10 万，世标发病率为 2.77/10 万；男性世标发病率为女性的 1.79 倍，城区世标发病率为郊区的 1.26 倍。0~74 岁累积发病率为 0.32%（表 5.1.1）。

5.1 Oral cavity & pharynx（C00-10, C12-14）

There were 769 new cases diagnosed as oral cavity and pharynx cancer（493 males and 276 females, 531 in urban areas and 238 in peri-urban areas）, accounting for 1.32% of new cases of all cancers in 2019. Oral cavity and pharynx cancer was the 18th common cancer in Beijing. The crude incidence rate was 5.55 per 100,000, with an ASR China and an ASR World of 2.84 and 2.77 per 100,000, respectively. The incidence of ASR World were 79% higher in males than in females and 26% higher in urban areas than in peri-urban areas. The cumulative incidence rate for subjects aged 0 to 74 years was 0.32%（Table 5.1.1）.

表 5.1.1 2019 年北京市户籍居民口腔癌和咽癌发病情况
Table 5.1.1 Incidence of oral cavity and pharynx cancer in Beijing, 2019

地区 Area	性别 Sex	例数 No. of cases	粗率 Crude rate （1/10^5）	构成比 Freq.（%）	中标率 ASR China （1/10^5）	世标率 ASR World （1/10^5）	累积率 Cumulative rate（0~74, %）	顺位 Rank
全市 All areas	合计 Both	769	5.55	1.32	2.84	2.77	0.32	18
	男性 Male	493	7.15	1.73	3.58	3.57	0.43	14
	女性 Female	276	3.96	0.93	2.12	1.99	0.20	17
城区 Urban areas	合计 Both	531	6.22	1.39	3.06	2.99	0.34	17
	男性 Male	330	7.78	1.78	3.76	3.76	0.45	14
	女性 Female	201	4.67	1.03	2.37	2.24	0.23	17
郊区 Peri-urban areas	合计 Both	238	4.47	1.18	2.46	2.38	0.28	19
	男性 Male	163	6.14	1.62	3.29	3.25	0.40	14
	女性 Female	75	2.81	0.74	1.68	1.55	0.17	18

2019 年，北京市口腔癌和咽癌死亡病例数为 363 例，占全部恶性肿瘤死亡的 1.33%，位居恶性肿瘤死亡第 16 位；其中男性 265 例，女性 98 例，城区 239 例，郊区 124 例。口腔癌和咽癌死亡率为 2.62/10 万，中标死亡率为 1.10/10 万，世标死亡率为 1.11/10 万；男性世标死亡率为女性的 3.46 倍，城区世标死亡率与郊区相近。0~74 岁累积死亡率为 0.13%（表 5.1.2）。

A total of 363 cases died of oral cavity and pharynx cancer（265 males and 98 females, 239 in urban areas and 124 in peri-urban areas）, accounting for 1.33% of all cancer deaths in 2019. Oral cavity and pharynx cancer was the 16th leading cause of cancer deaths in all cancers. The crude mortality rate was 2.62 per 100,000, with an ASR China and an ASR World of 1.10 and 1.11 per 100,000, respectively. The ASR World for mortality was 246% higher in males than in females, and that was similar in urban areas and in peri-urban areas. The cumulative mortality rate for subjects aged 0 to 74 years was 0.13%（Table 5.1.2）.

表 5.1.2 2019 年北京市户籍居民口腔癌和咽癌死亡情况
Table 5.1.2 Mortality of oral cavity and pharynx cancer in Beijing, 2019

地区 Area	性别 Sex	例数 No. of deaths	粗率 Crude rate（1/10^5）	构成比 Freq.（%）	中标率 ASR China（1/10^5）	世标率 ASR World（1/10^5）	累积率 Cumulative rate（0~74, %）	顺位 Rank
全市 All areas	合计 Both	363	2.62	1.33	1.10	1.11	0.13	16
	男性 Male	265	3.84	1.64	1.69	1.74	0.21	14
	女性 Female	98	1.41	0.88	0.53	0.50	0.05	17
城区 Urban areas	合计 Both	239	2.80	1.34	1.11	1.11	0.12	16
	男性 Male	169	3.98	1.63	1.68	1.71	0.20	14
	女性 Female	70	1.63	0.94	0.56	0.54	0.05	17
郊区 Peri-urban areas	合计 Both	124	2.33	1.30	1.07	1.10	0.13	16
	男性 Male	96	3.62	1.64	1.72	1.82	0.23	14
	女性 Female	28	1.05	0.76	0.46	0.44	0.05	17

北京市口腔癌和咽癌世标发病率由 2010 年的 2.17/10 万上升到 2019 年的 2.77/10 万，年均变化百分比（annual percentage change, APC）为 1.70%（P = 0.008）；男性和女性世标发病率 10 年间年均变化百分比分别为 1.90%（P = 0.016）和 1.40%（P = 0.104）。北京市口腔癌和咽癌世标死亡率由 2010 年的 0.98/10 万上升到

The incidence of ASR World of oral cavity and pharynx cancer increased from 2.17 per 100,000 in 2010 to 2.77 per 100,000 in 2019; and the APC of ASR World for incidence was 1.70%（P = 0.008）. The APCs of ASR World for incidence of oral cavity and pharynx cancer in males and females were 1.90%（P = 0.016）and 1.40%（P = 0.104）, respectively. The mortality of ASR World of oral cavity and pharynx cancer increased from 0.98 per 100,000 in 2010 to 1.11 per 100,000 in 2019; and the APC of ASR World for mortality was 1.84%（P < 0.001）. The APCs of ASR

2019 年的 1.11/10 万，年均变化百分比为 1.84%（$P < 0.001$）；男性和女性世标死亡率 10 年间年均变化百分比分别为 2.39%（$P = 0.002$）和 0.55%（$P = 0.729$）。

口腔癌和咽癌年龄别发病率和死亡率在 45 岁以前均较低，45 岁以后快速上升，男性上升速度高于女性（图 5.1.1 至图 5.1.6）。除 85 岁及以上年龄组女性发病率高于男性外，45 岁以上年龄组男性口腔癌和咽癌发病率及死亡率均高于女性。男性和女性发病率均在 75～79 岁组达到高峰，死亡率均在 85 岁及以上年龄组达到高峰（图 5.1.1 和图 5.1.4）。城区和郊区年龄别发病率、死亡率变化存在一定差异，但总体趋势相同（图 5.1.2 和图 5.1.3，图 5.1.5 和图 5.1.6）。

World for mortality of oral cavity and pharynx cancer in males and females were 2.39%（$P = 0.002$）and 0.55%（$P = 0.729$）, respectively.

The age-specific incidence and mortality rates of oral cavity and pharynx cancer were relatively low in people below 45 years old, and the rates increased sharply in people older than that, and the growth rates were higher in males than in females（Figure 5.1.1-5.1.6）. Except the incidence rate was higher in females than that in males at the age group of 85 years and above, the incidence and mortality rates in males were consistently higher than those in females after 45 years old. The age-specific incidence rates for both males and females peaked at the age group of 75-79 years. The age-specific mortality rates for both males and females peaked at the age group of 85 years and above（Figure 5.1.1, Figure 5.1.4）. There were some differences in age-specific incidence and mortality rates between urban and peri-urban areas, but the overall trends were same（Figure 5.1.2-5.1.3, Figure 5.1.5-5.1.6）.

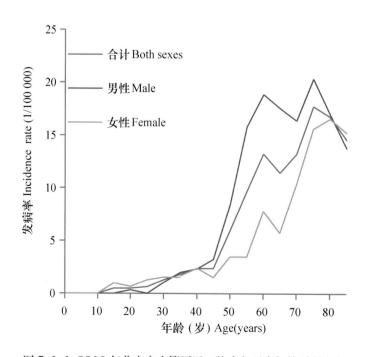

图 5.1.1 2019 年北京市户籍居民口腔癌和咽癌年龄别发病率

Figure 5.1.1 Age-specific incidence rates of oral cavity and pharynx cancer in Beijing, 2019

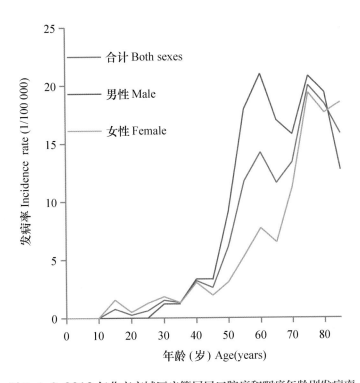

图 5.1.2 2019 年北京市城区户籍居民口腔癌和咽癌年龄别发病率
Figure 5.1.2 Age-specific incidence rates of oral cavity and pharynx cancer in urban areas of Beijing, 2019

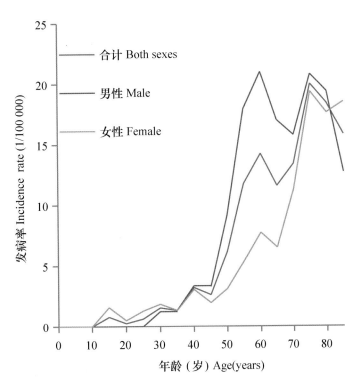

图 5.1.3 2019 年北京市郊区户籍居民口腔癌和咽癌年龄别发病率
Figure 5.1.3 Age-specific incidence rates of oral cavity and pharynx cancer in peri-urban areas of Beijing, 2019

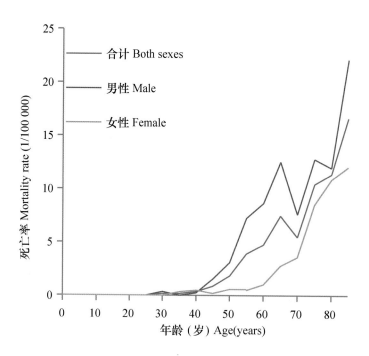

图 5.1.4 2019 年北京市户籍居民口腔癌和咽癌年龄别死亡率
Figure 5.1.4 Age-specific mortality rates of oral cavity and pharynx cancer in Beijing, 2019

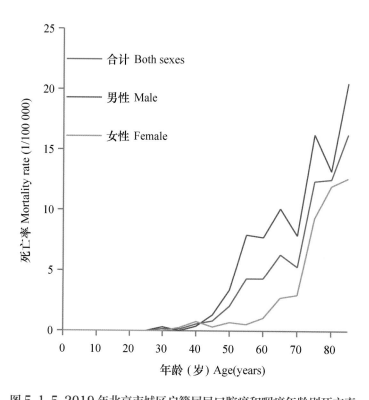

图 5.1.5 2019 年北京市城区户籍居民口腔癌和咽癌年龄别死亡率
Figure 5.1.5 Age-specific mortality rates of oral cavity and pharynx cancer in urban areas of Beijing, 2019

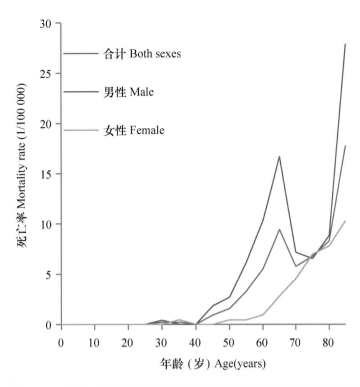

图 5.1.6 2019 年北京市郊区户籍居民口腔癌和咽癌年龄别死亡率
Figure 5.1.6 Age-specific mortality rates of oral cavity and pharynx cancer in peri-urban areas of Beijing, 2019

全部口腔癌和咽癌新发病例中，有明确亚部位的病例占 97.40%。其中，口腔是最常见的发病部位，占 32.51%；其后依次为舌、唾液腺和下咽，分别占 24.84%、15.35% 和 11.44%（图 5.1.7）。

About 97.40% of new cases were assigned to specified categories of oral cavity and pharynx cancer site. Among those, the mouth was the most common site, accounting for 32.51% of all cases, followed by the tongue（24.84%）, the salivary glands（15.35%）and the hypopharynx（11.44%）（Figure 5.1.7）.

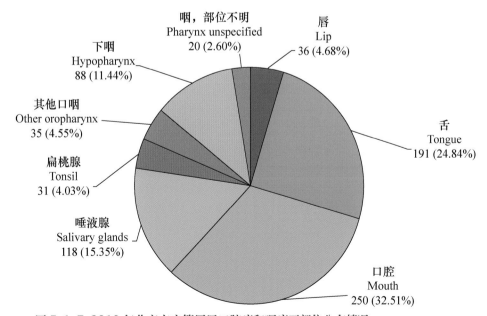

图 5.1.7 2019 年北京市户籍居民口腔癌和咽癌亚部位分布情况
Figure 5.1.7 Subsite distribution of oral cavity and pharynx cancer in Beijing, 2019

（撰稿 刘硕，校稿 李浩鑫）

5.2 鼻咽（C11）[1]

2019 年，北京市鼻咽癌新发病例数为 93 例，占全部恶性肿瘤发病的 0.16%，位居恶性肿瘤发病第 24 位；其中男性 64 例，女性 29 例，城区 65 例，郊区 28 例。鼻咽癌发病率为 0.67/10 万，中标发病率为 0.42/10 万，世标发病率为 0.39/10 万；男性世标发病率为女性的 2.74 倍，城区世标发病率为郊区的 1.33 倍。0~74 岁累积发病率为 0.04%（表 5.2.1）。

5.2 Nasopharynx（C11）[2]

There were 93 new cases diagnosed as nasopharyngeal cancer（64 males and 29 females, 65 in urban areas and 28 in peri-urban areas）, accounting for 0.16% of new cases of all cancers in 2019. Nasopharyngeal cancer was the 24th common cancer in Beijing. The crude incidence rate was 0.67 per 100,000, with an ASR China and an ASR World of 0.42 and 0.39 per 100,000, respectively. The ASR World for incidence was 174% higher in males than in females and 33% higher in urban areas than in peri-urban areas. The cumulative incidence rate for subjects aged 0 to 74 years was 0.04%（Table 5.2.1）.

表 5.2.1 2019 年北京市户籍居民鼻咽癌发病情况
Table 5.2.1 Incidence of nasopharyngeal cancer in Beijing, 2019

地区 Area	性别 Sex	例数 No. of cases	粗率 Crude rate （1/10^5）	构成比 Freq.（%）	中标率 ASR China （1/10^5）	世标率 ASR World （1/10^5）	累积率 Cumulative rate（0~74, %）	顺位 Rank
全市 All areas	合计 Both	93	0.67	0.16	0.42	0.39	0.04	24
	男性 Male	64	0.93	0.22	0.61	0.58	0.06	19
	女性 Female	29	0.42	0.10	0.23	0.21	0.02	22
城区 Urban areas	合计 Both	65	0.76	0.17	0.47	0.44	0.05	24
	男性 Male	45	1.06	0.24	0.69	0.64	0.07	18
	女性 Female	20	0.46	0.10	0.26	0.24	0.03	22
郊区 Peri-urban areas	合计 Both	28	0.53	0.14	0.34	0.33	0.03	24
	男性 Male	19	0.72	0.19	0.50	0.48	0.04	20
	女性 Female	9	0.34	0.09	0.18	0.17	0.02	22

2019 年，北京市鼻咽癌死亡病例数为 88 例，占全部恶性肿瘤死亡的 0.32%，位居恶性肿瘤死亡第 23 位；其中男性 66 例，女性 22 例，城区 58

A total of 88 cases died of nasopharyngeal cancer（66 males and 22 females, 58 in urban areas and 30 in peri-urban areas）, accounting for 0.32% of all cancer deaths in 2019. Nasopharyngeal cancer was

---

[1] 因北京市鼻咽癌发病和死亡例数较少，本节不包含年龄别发病率和死亡率的统计数据及图表。

[2] Because of few nasopharyngeal cancer cases and deaths occurred in Beijing in 2019, this section does not contain statistical data and charts on age-specific incidence and mortality rates.

例，郊区 30 例。鼻咽癌死亡率为 0.63/10 万，中标死亡率为 0.33/10 万，世标死亡率为 0.31/10 万；男性世标死亡率为女性的 3.42 倍，城区与郊区世标死亡率均为 0.31/10 万。0~74 岁累积死亡率为 0.03%（表 5.2.2）。

the 23rd leading cause of cancer deaths in all cancers. The crude mortality rate was 0.63 per 100,000, with an ASR China and an ASR World of 0.33 and 0.31 per 100,000, respectively. The ASR World for mortality was 242% higher in males than in females. The ASR World for mortality of both urban and peri-urban areas were 0.31 per 100,000. The cumulative mortality rate for subjects aged 0 to 74 years was 0.03% (Table 5.2.2) .

表 5.2.2 2019 年北京市户籍居民鼻咽癌死亡情况
Table 5.2.2 Mortality of nasopharyngeal cancer in Beijing, 2019

地区 Area	性别 Sex	例数 No. of deaths	粗率 Crude rate （1/10⁵）	构成比 Freq.（%）	中标率 ASR China （1/10⁵）	世标率 ASR World （1/10⁵）	累积率 Cumulative rate（0~74, %）	顺位 Rank
全市 All areas	合计 Both	88	0.63	0.32	0.33	0.31	0.03	23
	男性 Male	66	0.96	0.41	0.51	0.49	0.05	17
	女性 Female	22	0.32	0.20	0.15	0.14	0.02	22
城区 Urban areas	合计 Both	58	0.68	0.32	0.33	0.31	0.04	22
	男性 Male	42	0.99	0.41	0.46	0.46	0.05	17
	女性 Female	16	0.37	0.21	0.20	0.18	0.02	22
郊区 Peri-urban areas	合计 Both	30	0.56	0.32	0.32	0.31	0.03	23
	男性 Male	24	0.90	0.41	0.57	0.54	0.04	17
	女性 Female	6	0.22	0.16	0.08	0.09	0.01	22

北京市鼻咽癌世标发病率由2010年的0.64/10万下降到2019年的0.39/10万，年均变化百分比为 -6.69%（$P=0.001$）；男性和女性世标发病率10年间年均变化百分比分别为 -6.13%（$P=0.001$）和 -7.91%（$P=0.006$）。北京市鼻咽癌的世标死亡率2010年为0.38/10万，2019年为0.31/10万，年均变化百分比为 -1.91%（$P=0.133$）；男性和女性世标死亡率10年间年均变化百分比分别为 -0.91%（$P=0.559$）和 -4.14%（$P=0.208$）。

The ASR World for incidence of nasopharyngeal cancer decreased from 0.64 per 100,000 in 2010 to 0.39 per 100,000 in 2019; and the APC of ASR World for incidence was -6.69% ($P=0.001$) . The APCs of ASR World for incidence of nasopharyngeal cancer in males and females were -6.13% ($P=0.001$) and -7.91% ($P=0.006$) , respectively. The ASR World for mortality of nasopharyngeal cancer was 0.38 per 100,000 in 2010, and 0.31 per 100,000 in 2019; and the APC of ASR World for mortality was -1.91% ($P=0.133$) . The APCs of ASR World for mortality of nasopharyngeal cancer in males and females were -0.91% ($P=0.559$) and -4.14% ($P=0.208$) , respectively.

（撰稿 刘硕，校稿 李慧超）

5.3 食管（C15）

2019 年，北京市食管癌新发病例数为 1 190 例，占全部恶性肿瘤发病的 2.04%，位居恶性肿瘤发病第 15 位；其中男性 933 例，女性 257 例，城区 653 例，郊区 537 例。食管癌发病率为 8.58/10 万，中标发病率为 3.50/10 万，世标发病率为 3.59/10 万；男性世标发病率为女性的 5.04 倍，郊区世标发病率为城区的 1.54 倍。0～74 岁累积发病率为 0.42%（表 5.3.1）。

5.3 Esophagus（C15）

There were 1,190 new cases diagnosed as esophageal cancer（933 males and 257 females, 653 in urban areas and 537 in peri-urban areas）, accounting for 2.04% of new cases of all cancers in 2019. Esophageal cancer was the 15th common cancer in Beijing. The crude incidence rate was 8.58 per 100,000, with an ASR China and an ASR World of 3.50 and 3.59 per 100,000, respectively. The ASR World for incidence was 404% higher in males than in females and 54% higher in peri-urban areas than in urban areas. The cumulative incidence rate for subjects aged 0 to 74 years was 0.42%（Table 5.3.1）.

表 5.3.1 2019 年北京市户籍居民食管癌发病情况
Table 5.3.1 Incidence of esophageal cancer in Beijing, 2019

地区 Area	性别 Sex	例数 No. of cases	粗率 Crude rate （1/10^5）	构成比 Freq.（%）	中标率 ASR China （1/10^5）	世标率 ASR World （1/10^5）	累积率 Cumulative rate（0~74, %）	顺位 Rank
全市 All areas	合计 Both	1 190	8.58	2.04	3.50	3.59	0.42	15
	男性 Male	933	13.53	3.27	5.97	6.11	0.73	9
	女性 Female	257	3.69	0.87	1.18	1.21	0.12	18
城区 Urban areas	合计 Both	653	7.64	1.72	2.89	3.01	0.35	15
	男性 Male	513	12.09	2.77	4.94	5.15	0.60	11
	女性 Female	140	3.25	0.72	0.94	0.96	0.10	18
郊区 Peri-urban areas	合计 Both	537	10.09	2.66	4.60	4.63	0.54	11
	男性 Male	420	15.83	4.17	7.73	7.73	0.93	9
	女性 Female	117	4.38	1.16	1.66	1.72	0.17	16

2019 年，北京市食管癌死亡病例数为 1 008 例，占全部恶性肿瘤死亡的 3.69%，位居恶性肿瘤死亡第 9 位；其中男性 805 例，女性 203 例，城区

A total of 1,008 cases died of esophageal cancer（805 males and 203 females, 556 in urban areas and 452 in peri-urban areas）, accounting for 3.69% of all cancer deaths in 2019. Esophageal

556 例，郊区 452 例。食管癌死亡率为 7.27/10 万，中标死亡率为 2.80/10 万，世标死亡率为 2.87/10 万；男性世标死亡率为女性的 5.77 倍，郊区世标死亡率为城区的 1.61 倍。0~74 岁累积死亡率为 0.31%（表 5.3.2）。

cancer was the 9th leading cause of cancer deaths in all cancers. The crude mortality rate was 7.27 per 100,000, with an ASR China and an ASR World of 2.80 and 2.87 per 100,000, respectively. The ASR World for mortality was 477% higher in males than in females and 61% higher in peri-urban areas than in urban areas. The cumulative mortality rate for subjects aged 0 to 74 years was 0.31%（Table 5.3.2）.

表 5.3.2 2019 年北京市户籍居民食管癌死亡情况
Table 5.3.2 Mortality of esophageal cancer in Beijing, 2019

地区 Area	性别 Sex	例数 No. of deaths	粗率 Crude rate（1/10⁵）	构成比 Freq.（%）	中标率 ASR China（1/10⁵）	世标率 ASR World（1/10⁵）	累积率 Cumulative rate（0~74, %）	顺位 Rank
全市 All areas	合计 Both	1 008	7.27	3.69	2.80	2.87	0.31	9
	男性 Male	805	11.68	4.97	4.91	5.02	0.58	5
	女性 Female	203	2.91	1.82	0.84	0.87	0.06	15
城区 Urban areas	合计 Both	556	6.51	3.12	2.25	2.35	0.25	11
	男性 Male	439	10.35	4.23	3.94	4.10	0.46	7
	女性 Female	117	2.72	1.56	0.67	0.70	0.04	16
郊区 Peri-urban areas	合计 Both	452	8.49	4.76	3.79	3.79	0.42	5
	男性 Male	366	13.80	6.27	6.60	6.58	0.77	5
	女性 Female	86	3.22	2.35	1.19	1.21	0.09	13

北京市食管癌世标发病率由 2010 年的 5.29/10 万下降到 2019 年的 3.59/10 万，年均变化百分比为 −4.42%（$P < 0.001$）；男性和女性世标发病率 10 年间年均变化百分比分别为 −3.93%（$P < 0.001$）和 −6.71%（$P < 0.001$）。北京市食管癌世标死亡率由 2010 年的 4.26/10 万下

The ASR World for incidence of esophageal cancer decreased from 5.29 per 100,000 in 2010 to 3.59 per 100,000 in 2019; and the APC of ASR World for incidence was −4.42%（$P < 0.001$）. The APCs of ASR World for incidence of esophageal cancer in males and females were −3.93%（$P < 0.001$）and −6.71%（$P < 0.001$）, respectively. The ASR World for mortality of esophageal cancer decreased from 4.26 per 100,000 in 2010 to 2.87 per 100,000 in 2019; and the APC of

降到 2019 年的 2.87/10 万，年均变化百分比为 -4.38%（$P < 0.001$）；男性和女性世标死亡率 10 年间年均变化百分比分别为 -3.89%（$P < 0.001$）和 -6.45%（$P < 0.001$）。

食管癌年龄别发病率和死亡率在 40 岁以前均较低，40 岁以后快速上升，男性上升速度高于女性（图 5.3.1 至图 5.3.6）。40 岁以上年龄组男性食管癌发病率和死亡率均高于女性，男性和女性发病率和死亡率均在 85 岁及以上年龄组达到高峰（图 5.3.1 和图 5.3.4）。城区和郊区年龄别发病率、死亡率变化存在差异，但总体趋势相同（图 5.3.2 和图 5.3.3，图 5.3.5 和图 5.3.6）。

ASR World for mortality was -4.38%（$P < 0.001$）. The APCs of ASR World for mortality of esophageal cancer in males and females were -3.89%（$P < 0.001$）and -6.45%（$P < 0.001$）, respectively.

The age-specific incidence and mortality rates of esophageal cancer were relatively low in people below 40 years old, but the rates increased sharply in people older than that; furthermore, the growth rates were higher in males than those in females（Figure 5.3.1-5.3.6）. The incidence and mortality rates in males were consistently higher than those in females after 40 years old, and the age-specific incidence and mortality rates for both sexes peaked at the age group of 85 years and above（Figure 5.3.1, Figure 5.3.4）. There were some differences in age-specific incidence and mortality rates between urban and peri-urban areas, but the overall trends were same（Figure 5.3.2-5.3.3, Figure 5.3.5-5.3.6）.

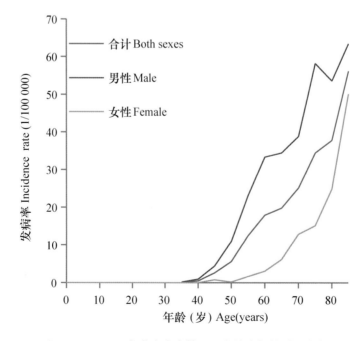

图 5.3.1 2019 年北京市户籍居民食管癌年龄别发病率
Figure 5.3.1 Age-specific incidence rates of esophageal cancer in Beijing, 2019

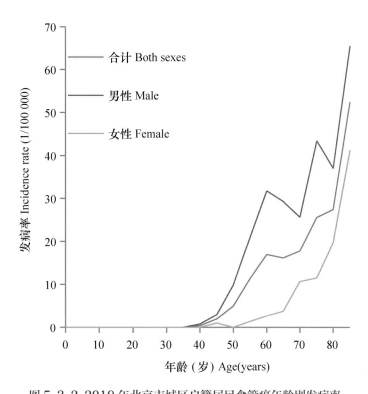

图 5.3.2 2019 年北京市城区户籍居民食管癌年龄别发病率
Figure 5.3.2 Age-specific incidence rates of esophageal cancer in urban areas of Beijing, 2019

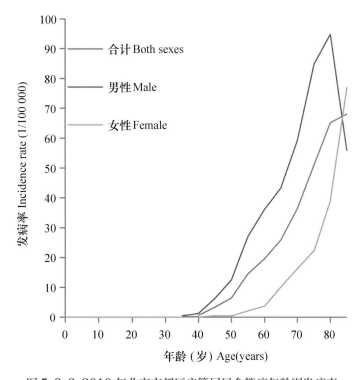

图 5.3.3 2019 年北京市郊区户籍居民食管癌年龄别发病率
Figure 5.3.3 Age-specific incidence rates of esophageal cancer in peri-urban areas of Beijing, 2019

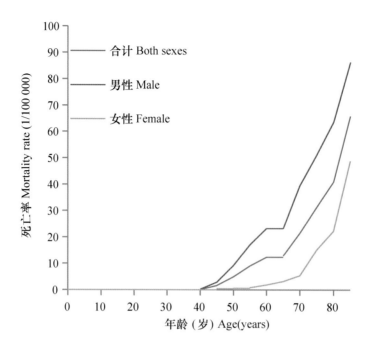

图 5.3.4 2019 年北京市户籍居民食管癌年龄别死亡率
Figure 5.3.4 Age-specific mortality rates of esophageal cancer in Beijing, 2019

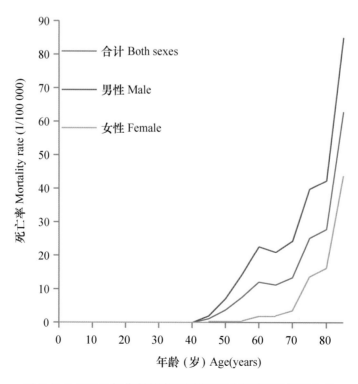

图 5.3.5 2019 年北京市城区户籍居民食管癌年龄别死亡率
Figure 5.3.5 Age-specific mortality rates of esophageal cancer in urban areas of Beijing, 2019

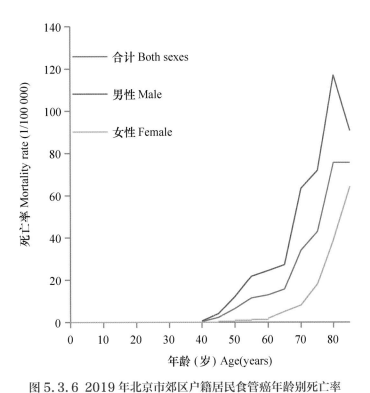

图 5.3.6 2019 年北京市郊区户籍居民食管癌年龄别死亡率
Figure 5.3.6 Age-specific mortality rates of esophageal cancer in peri-urban areas of Beijing, 2019

2019 年，北京市食管癌世标发病率和死亡率在 16 个辖区间存在显著差异，郊区发病率和死亡率均高于城区（图 5.3.7 和图 5.3.8）。

In 2019, there were significant differences among the 16 districts in ASR World for incidence and mortality of esophageal cancer in Beijing. The incidence and mortality rates were higher in peri-urban areas than in urban areas (Figure 5.3.7-5.3.8).

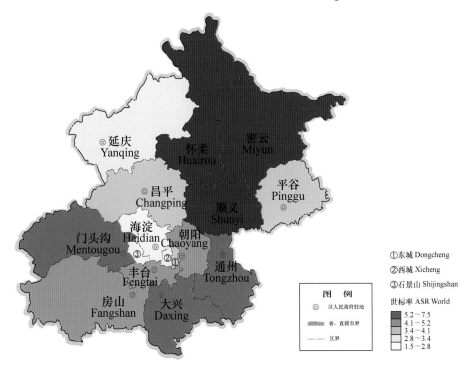

图 5.3.7 2019 年北京市户籍居民食管癌世标发病率（1/10⁵）地区分布情况
Figure 5.3.7 ASRs World for incidence of esophageal cancer（1/10⁵）by district in Beijing, 2019

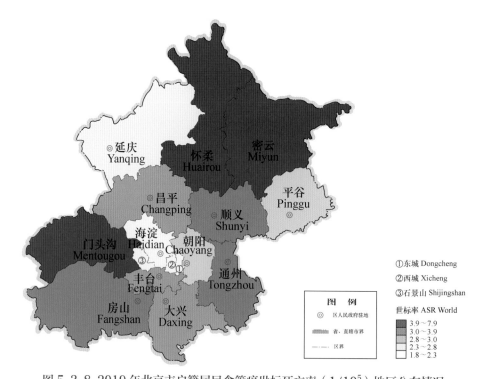

图 5.3.8 2019 年北京市户籍居民食管癌世标死亡率（1/10⁵）地区分布情况
Figure 5.3.8 ASRs World for mortality of esophageal cancer（1/10⁵）by district in Beijing, 2019

全部食管癌新发病例中，有明确亚部位的病例占 44.37%。其中食管中三分之一是最常见的发病部位，占 84.09%；其后依次为食管下三之分一、交搭跨越、食管上三之分一，分别占 7.20%、5.30% 和 3.41%（图 5.3.9）。

About 44.37% of new cases were assigned to specified categories of esophageal cancer site. Among those, the middle third of the esophagus was the most common site, accounting for 84.09% of all cases, followed by the lower third of the esophagus（7.20%）, the overlapping（5.30%）and the upper third of the esophagus（3.41%）（Figure 5.3.9）.

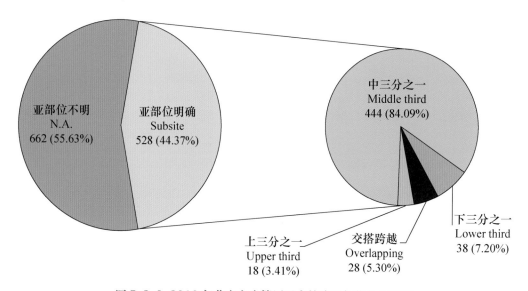

图 5.3.9 2019 年北京市户籍居民食管癌亚部位分布情况
Figure 5.3.9 Subsite distribution of esophageal cancer in Beijing, 2019

（撰稿 李浩鑫，校稿 张希）

5.4 胃（C16）

2019 年，北京市胃癌新发病例数为 2 635 例，占全部恶性肿瘤发病的 4.52%，位居恶性肿瘤发病第 5 位；其中男性 1 820 例，女性 815 例，城区 1 808 例，郊区 827 例。胃癌发病率为 19.00/10 万，中标发病率为 8.36/10 万，世标发病率为 8.23/10 万；男性世标发病率为女性的 2.35 倍，城区世标发病率为郊区的 1.17 倍。0~74 岁累积发病率为 0.95%（表 5.4.1）。

5.4 Stomach（C16）

There were 2,635 new cases diagnosed as stomach cancer (1,820 males and 815 females, 1,808 in urban areas and 827 in peri-urban areas), accounting for 4.52% of new cases of all cancers in 2019. Stomach cancer was the 5th common cancer in Beijing. The crude incidence rate was 19.00 per 100,000, with an ASR China and an ASR World of 8.36 and 8.23 per 100,000, respectively. The ASR World for incidence was 135% higher in males than in females and 17% higher in urban areas than in peri-urban areas. The cumulative incidence rate for subjects aged 0 to 74 years was 0.95% (Table 5.4.1).

表 5.4.1 2019 年北京市户籍居民胃癌发病情况
Table 5.4.1 Incidence of stomach cancer in Beijing, 2019

地区 Area	性别 Sex	例数 No. of cases	粗率 Crude rate （1/10⁵）	构成比 Freq.（%）	中标率 ASR China （1/10⁵）	世标率 ASR World （1/10⁵）	累积率 Cumulative rate（0~74, %）	顺位 Rank
全市 All areas	合计 Both	2 635	19.00	4.52	8.36	8.23	0.95	5
	男性 Male	1 820	26.40	6.37	11.82	11.75	1.39	3
	女性 Female	815	11.69	2.75	5.21	5.00	0.54	8
城区 Urban areas	合计 Both	1 808	21.16	4.75	8.81	8.67	1.01	5
	男性 Male	1 220	28.76	6.60	12.08	12.03	1.45	4
	女性 Female	588	13.67	3.00	5.85	5.60	0.60	7
郊区 Peri-urban areas	合计 Both	827	15.54	4.10	7.58	7.43	0.85	6
	男性 Male	600	22.62	5.96	11.33	11.23	1.29	5
	女性 Female	227	8.50	2.25	4.14	3.96	0.44	11

2019年，北京市胃癌死亡病例数为1 907例，占全部恶性肿瘤死亡的6.97%，位居恶性肿瘤死亡第4位；其中男性1 307例，女性600例，城区1 295例，郊区612例。胃癌死亡率为13.75/10万，中标死亡率为5.39/10万，世标死亡率为5.32/10万；男性世标死亡率为女性的2.34倍，城区世标死亡率为郊区的1.02倍。0~74岁累积死亡率为0.56%（表5.4.2）。

A total of 1,907 cases died of stomach cancer（1,307 males and 600 females, 1,295 in urban areas and 612 in peri-urban areas）, accounting for 6.97% of all cancer deaths in 2019. Stomach cancer was the 4th leading cause of cancer deaths in all cancers. The crude mortality rate was 13.75 per 100,000, with an ASR China and an ASR World of 5.39 and 5.32 per 100,000, respectively. The ASR World for mortality was 134% higher in males than in females and 2% higher in urban areas than in peri-urban areas. The cumulative mortality rate for subjects aged 0 to 74 years was 0.56%（Table 5.4.2）.

表5.4.2 2019年北京市户籍居民胃癌死亡情况
Table 5.4.2 Mortality of stomach cancer in Beijing, 2019

地区 Area	性别 Sex	例数 No. of deaths	粗率 Crude rate （1/10⁵）	构成比 Freq.（%）	中标率 ASR China （1/10⁵）	世标率 ASR World （1/10⁵）	累积率 Cumulative rate（0~74, %）	顺位 Rank
全市 All areas	合计 Both	1 907	13.75	6.97	5.39	5.32	0.56	4
	男性 Male	1 307	18.96	8.07	7.64	7.64	0.84	4
	女性 Female	600	8.61	5.38	3.39	3.26	0.31	5
城区 Urban areas	合计 Both	1 295	15.16	7.26	5.38	5.34	0.56	3
	男性 Male	874	20.60	8.43	7.49	7.52	0.82	3
	女性 Female	421	9.79	5.63	3.51	3.39	0.32	5
郊区 Peri-urban areas	合计 Both	612	11.50	6.44	5.34	5.22	0.56	4
	男性 Male	433	16.32	7.42	7.79	7.72	0.87	4
	女性 Female	179	6.70	4.88	3.17	3.00	0.28	7

北京市胃癌世标发病率由2010年的9.96/10万下降到2019年的8.23/10万，年均变化百分比为-2.38%（ $P < 0.001$ ）；男性和女性世标发病率10年间年均变化百分比分别为-2.06%

The ASR World for incidence of stomach cancer decreased from 9.96 per 100,000 in 2010 to 8.23 per 100,000 in 2019; and the APC of ASR World for incidence was -2.38%（ $P < 0.001$ ）. The APCs of ASR World for incidence of stomach cancer in males and females were -2.06%（ $P < 0.001$ ）and -2.91%

（P < 0.001）和 -2.91%（P < 0.001）。北京市胃癌世标死亡率由2010年的6.80/10万下降到2019年的5.32/10万，年均变化百分比为 -2.92%（P < 0.001）；男性和女性世标死亡率10年间年均变化百分比分别为 -2.86%（P = 0.001）和 -2.81%（P < 0.001）。

胃癌年龄别发病率和死亡率在45岁以前均较低，45岁以后快速上升，男性上升速度高于女性（图 5.4.1 至图 5.4.6）。男性发病率在80~84岁组达到高峰，男性死亡率以及女性发病率和死亡率均在85岁及以上年龄组达到高峰（图 5.4.1 和图 5.4.4）。城区和郊区年龄别发病率、死亡率变化有一定差异，但总体趋势相同（图 5.4.2 和图 5.4.3，图 5.4.5 和图 5.4.6）。

（P < 0.001）, respectively. The ASR World for mortality of stomach cancer decreased from 6.80 per 100,000 in 2010 to 5.32 per 100,000 in 2019; and the APC of ASR World for mortality was -2.92%（P < 0.001）. The APCs of ASR World for mortality of stomach cancer in males and females were -2.86%（P=0.001）and -2.81%（P < 0.001）, respectively.

The age-specific incidence and mortality rates of stomach cancer were relatively low in people below 45 years old, and the rates increased sharply in people older than that; furthermore, the growth rates were higher in males than in females（Figure 5.4.1-5.4.6）. The age-specific incidence rates for males peaked at the age group of 80-84 years. However, the age-specific mortality rates for both sexes and the incidence rates for females peaked at the age group of 85 years and above（Figure 5.4.1, Figure 5.4.4）. There were some differences in age-specific incidence and mortality rates between urban and peri-urban areas, but the overall trends were same（Figure 5.4.2-5.4.3, Figure 5.4.5-5.4.6）.

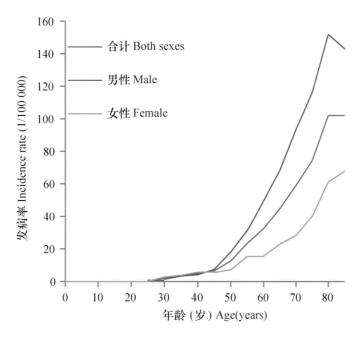

图 5.4.1　2019 年北京市户籍居民胃癌年龄别发病率
Figure 5.4.1 Age-specific incidence rates of stomach cancer in Beijing, 2019

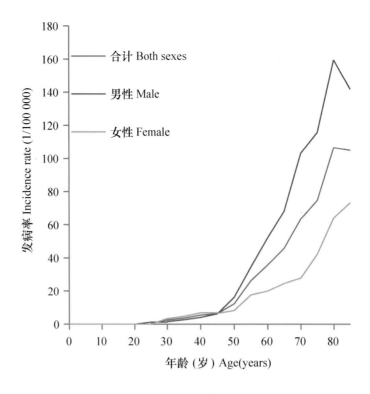

图 5.4.2 2019 年北京市城区户籍居民胃癌年龄别发病率
Figure 5.4.2 Age-specific incidence rates of stomach cancer in urban areas of Beijing, 2019

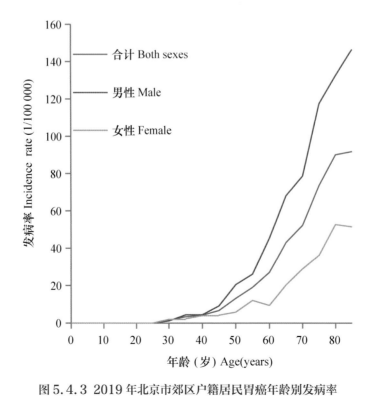

图 5.4.3 2019 年北京市郊区户籍居民胃癌年龄别发病率
Figure 5.4.3 Age-specific incidence rates of stomach cancer in peri-urban areas of Beijing, 2019

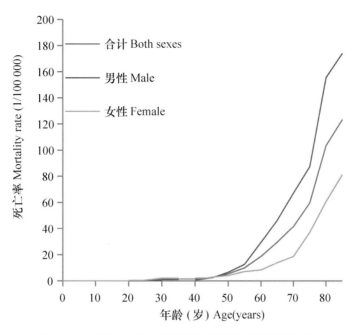

图 5.4.4 2019 年北京市户籍居民胃癌年龄别死亡率
Figure 5.4.4 Age-specific mortality rates of stomach cancer in Beijing, 2019

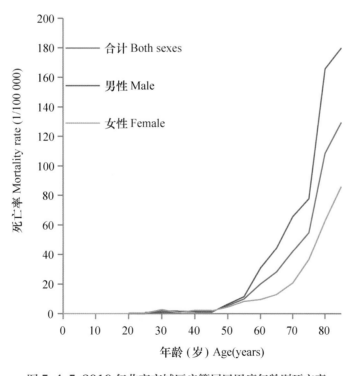

图 5.4.5 2019 年北京市城区户籍居民胃癌年龄别死亡率
Figure 5.4.5 Age-specific mortality rates of stomach cancer in urban areas of Beijing, 2019

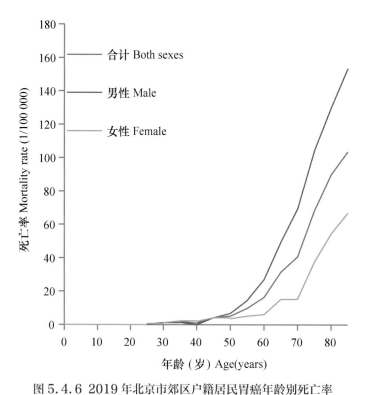

图 5.4.6 2019 年北京市郊区户籍居民胃癌年龄别死亡率
Figure 5.4.6 Age-specific mortality rates of stomach cancer in peri-urban areas of Beijing, 2019

2019 年，北京市胃癌世标发病率和死亡率在 16 个辖区间有一定差异，城区发病率和死亡率均高于郊区（图 5.4.7，图 5.4.8）。

In 2019, there were some differences among the 16 districts in ASR World for incidence and mortality of stomach cancer in Beijing. The incidence and mortality rates were higher in urban areas than in peri-urban areas（Figure 5.4.7-5.4.8）.

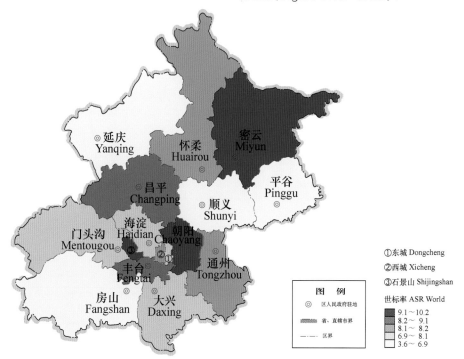

图 5.4.7 2019 年北京市户籍居民胃癌世标发病率（1/10⁵）地区分布情况
Figure 5.4.7 ASRs World for incidence of stomach cancer（$1/10^5$）by district in Beijing, 2019

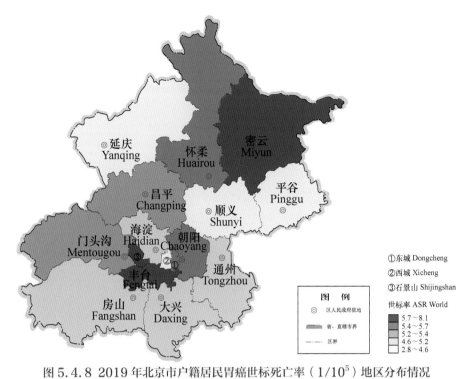

图 5.4.8 2019 年北京市户籍居民胃癌世标死亡率（1/10^5）地区分布情况
Figure 5.4.8 ASRs World for mortality mortality of stomach cancer（1/10^5）by district in Beijing, 2019

全部胃癌新发病例中，有明确亚部位的病例占 54.35%。其中幽门窦是最常见的发病部位，占 34.99%；其后依次为贲门（28.07%）、胃体（15.01%）、交搭跨越（7.33%）、胃小弯（6.63%）、胃底（5.59%）、幽门（1.19%）和胃大弯（1.19%）（图 5.4.9）。

About 54.35% of new cases were assigned to specified categories of stomach cancer site. Among those, the pyloric antrum was the most common subsite, accounting for 34.99% of all cases, followed by the cardia（28.07%）, the body（15.01%）, the overlapping（7.33%）, the lesser curvature（6.63%）, the fundus（5.59%）, the pylorus（1.19%）, and the greater curvature（1.19%）（Figure 5.4.9）.

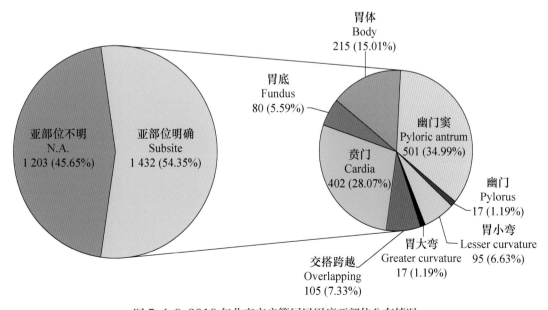

图 5.4.9 2019 年北京市户籍居民胃癌亚部位分布情况
Figure 5.4.9 Subsite distribution of stomach cancer in Beijing, 2019

（撰稿 杨雷，校稿 李晴雨）

5.5 结直肠（C18-21）

2019 年，北京市结直肠癌新发病例数为 7 349 例，占全部恶性肿瘤发病的 12.62%，位居恶性肿瘤发病第 2 位；其中男性 4 348 例，女性 3 001 例，城区 4 965 例，郊区 2 384 例。结直肠癌发病率为 53.00/10 万，中标发病率为 24.01/10 万，世标发病率为 23.73/10 万；男性世标发病率为女性的 1.58 倍，城区世标发病率为郊区的 1.12 倍。0~74 岁累积发病率为 2.85%（表 5.5.1）。

5.5 Colon-rectum（C18-21）

There were 7,349 new cases diagnosed as colorectal cancer（4,348 males and 3,001 females, 4,965 in urban areas and 2,384 in peri-urban areas）, accounting for 12.62% of new cases of all cancers in 2019. Colorectal cancer was the 2nd common cancer in Beijing. The crude incidence rate was 53.00 per 100,000, with an ASR China and an ASR World of 24.01 and 23.73 per 100,000, respectively. The ASR World for incidence was 58% higher in males than in females and 12% higher in urban areas than in peri-urban areas. The cumulative incidence rate for subjects aged 0 to 74 years was 2.85%（Table 5.5.1）.

表 5.5.1 2019 年北京市户籍居民结直肠癌发病情况
Table 5.5.1 Incidence of colorectal cancer in Beijing, 2019

地区 Area	性别 Sex	例数 No. of cases	粗率 Crude rate （1/10⁵）	构成比 Freq.（%）	中标率 ASR China （1/10⁵）	世标率 ASR World （1/10⁵）	累积率 Cumulative rate（0~74, %）	顺位 Rank
全市 All areas	合计 Both	7 349	53.00	12.62	24.01	23.73	2.85	2
	男性 Male	4 348	63.06	15.22	29.35	29.25	3.57	2
	女性 Female	3 001	43.05	10.12	19.02	18.56	2.17	4
城区 Urban areas	合计 Both	4 965	58.12	13.04	24.97	24.69	2.99	2
	男性 Male	2 939	69.29	15.89	30.72	30.56	3.77	2
	女性 Female	2 026	47.10	10.35	19.56	19.14	2.25	4
郊区 Peri-urban areas	合计 Both	2 384	44.79	11.82	22.31	22.05	2.61	2
	男性 Male	1 409	53.12	13.99	27.00	27.03	3.23	2
	女性 Female	975	36.51	9.66	17.98	17.46	2.04	4

2019 年，北京市结直肠癌死亡病例数为 3 162 例，占全部恶性肿瘤死亡的 11.56%，位居恶性肿瘤死亡第 2 位；其中男性 1 812 例，女性 1 350 例，城区 2 218 例，郊区 944 例。结直肠癌死亡率为 22.80/10 万，中标死亡率为 8.46/10 万，世标死亡率为 8.39/10 万；男性世标死亡率为女性的 1.59 倍，城区世标死亡率为郊区的 1.11 倍。0~74 岁累积死亡率为 0.78%（表 5.5.2）。

A total of 3,162 cases died of colorectal cancer (1,812 males and 1,350 females, 2,218 in urban areas and 944 in peri-urban areas), accounting for 11.56% of all cancer deaths in 2019. Colorectal cancer was the 2nd leading cause of cancer deaths in all cancers. The crude mortality rate was 22.80 per 100,000, with an ASR China and an ASR World of 8.46 and 8.39 per 100,000, respectively. The ASR World for mortality was 59% higher in males than in females and 11% higher in urban areas than in peri-urban areas. The cumulative mortality rate for subjects aged 0 to 74 years was 0.78%(Table 5.5.2).

表 5.5.2 2019 年北京市户籍居民结直肠癌死亡情况
Table 5.5.2 Mortality of colorectal cancer in Beijing, 2019

地区 Area	性别 Sex	例数 No. of deaths	粗率 Crude rate （1/10⁵）	构成比 Freq.（%）	中标率 ASR China （1/10⁵）	世标率 ASR World （1/10⁵）	累积率 Cumulative rate（0~74, %）	顺位 Rank
全市 All areas	合计 Both	3 162	22.80	11.56	8.46	8.39	0.78	2
	男性 Male	1 812	26.28	11.18	10.50	10.41	1.02	2
	女性 Female	1 350	19.36	12.11	6.61	6.56	0.56	2
城区 Urban areas	合计 Both	2 218	25.96	12.43	8.75	8.71	0.84	2
	男性 Male	1 243	29.30	11.99	10.71	10.67	1.11	2
	女性 Female	975	22.67	13.03	6.95	6.91	0.60	2
郊区 Peri-urban areas	合计 Both	944	17.73	9.93	7.96	7.82	0.69	2
	男性 Male	569	21.45	9.75	10.21	9.99	0.88	3
	女性 Female	375	14.04	10.23	5.94	5.88	0.51	2

2019 年，北京市结肠癌（C18）新发病例数为 4 261 例，占全部恶性肿瘤发病的 7.32%；其中男性 2 392 例，女性 1 869 例，城区 3 015 例，郊区 1 246 例。结肠癌（C18）发病率为 30.73/10 万，中标发病率为 13.68/10 万，世标发病率为 13.47/10 万；男性世标发病率为女性的 1.41 倍，城区世标发病率为郊区的 1.26 倍。0~74 岁累积发病率为 1.57%（表 5.5.3）。

There were 4,261 new cases diagnosed as colon cancer（C18; 2,392 males and 1,869 females, 3,015 in urban areas and 1,246 in peri-urban areas）, accounting for 7.32% of new cases of all cancers in 2019. The crude incidence rate was 30.73 per 100,000, with an ASR China and an ASR World of 13.68 and 13.47 per 100,000, respectively. The ASR World for incidence was 41% higher in males than in females and 26% higher in urban areas than in peri-urban areas. The cumulative incidence rate for subjects aged 0 to 74 years was 1.57%（Table 5.5.3）.

表 5.5.3 2019 年北京市户籍居民结肠癌（C18）发病情况
Table 5.5.3 Incidence of colon cancer （C18） in Beijing, 2019

地区 Area	性别 Sex	例数 No. of cases	粗率 Crude rate （1/10^5）	构成比 Freq.（%）	中标率 ASR China （1/10^5）	世标率 ASR World （1/10^5）	累积率 Cumulative rate（0~74, %）
全市 All areas	合计 Both	4 261	30.73	7.32	13.68	13.47	1.57
	男性 Male	2 392	34.69	8.37	16.01	15.86	1.90
	女性 Female	1 869	26.81	6.30	11.51	11.22	1.27
城区 Urban areas	合计 Both	3 015	35.29	7.92	14.77	14.55	1.71
	男性 Male	1 700	40.08	9.19	17.49	17.29	2.08
	女性 Female	1 315	30.57	6.72	12.24	11.98	1.35
郊区 Peri-urban areas	合计 Both	1 246	23.41	6.18	11.74	11.52	1.36
	男性 Male	692	26.09	6.87	13.43	13.35	1.59
	女性 Female	554	20.75	5.49	10.17	9.83	1.14

2019 年，北京市结肠癌（C18）死亡病例数为 1 836 例，占全部恶性肿瘤死亡的 6.71%；其中男性 996 例，女性 840 例，城区 1 357 例，郊区 479 例。结肠癌（C18）死亡率为 13.24/10 万，中标死亡率为 4.80/10 万，世标死亡率为 4.73/10 万；男性世标死亡率为女性的 1.44 倍，城区世标死亡率为郊区的 1.30 倍。0~74 岁累积死亡率为 0.42%（表 5.5.4）。

A total of 1,836 cases died of colon cancer（C18; 996 males and 840 females, 1,357 in urban areas and 479 in peri-urban areas）, accounting for 6.71% of all cancer deaths in 2019. The crude mortality rate was 13.24 per 100,000, with an ASR China and an ASR World of 4.80 and 4.73 per 100,000, respectively. The ASR World for mortality was 44% higher in males than in females and 30% higher in urban areas than in peri-urban areas. The cumulative mortality rate for subjects aged 0 to 74 years was 0.42%（Table 5.5.4）.

表 5.5.4 2019 年北京市户籍居民结肠癌（C18）死亡情况
Table 5.5.4 Mortality of colon cancer （C18） in Beijing, 2019

地区 Area	性别 Sex	例数 No. of deaths	粗率 Crude rate （1/10^5）	构成比 Freq.（%）	中标率 ASR China （1/10^5）	世标率 ASR World （1/10^5）	累积率 Cumulative rate(0~74, %)
全市 All areas	合计 Both	1 836	13.24	6.71	4.80	4.73	0.42
	男性 Male	996	14.45	6.15	5.71	5.63	0.53
	女性 Female	840	12.05	7.54	3.97	3.90	0.31
城区 Urban areas	合计 Both	1 357	15.88	7.60	5.17	5.13	0.47
	男性 Male	719	16.95	6.94	6.07	6.02	0.60
	女性 Female	638	14.83	8.53	4.34	4.29	0.35
郊区 Peri-urban areas	合计 Both	479	9.00	5.04	4.09	3.94	0.33
	男性 Male	277	10.44	4.75	5.05	4.86	0.42
	女性 Female	202	7.56	5.51	3.22	3.12	0.25

2019 年，北京市直肠癌（C19-20）新发病例数为 3 061 例，占全部恶性肿瘤发病的 5.26%；其中男性 1 940 例，女性 1 121 例，城区 1 933 例，郊区 1 128 例。直肠癌（C19-20）发病率为 22.08/10 万，中标发病率为 10.21/10 万，世标发病率为 10.16/10 万；男性世标发病率为女性的 1.83 倍，郊区世标发病率为城区的 1.04 倍。0～74 岁累积发病率为 1.27%（表 5.5.5）。

There were 3,061 new cases diagnosed as rectal cancer（C19-20; 1,940 males and 1,121 females, 1,933 in urban areas and 1,128 in peri-urban areas）, accounting for 5.26% of new cases of all cancers in 2019. The crude incidence rate was 22.08 per 100,000, with an ASR China and an ASR World of 10.21 and 10.16 per 100,000, respectively. The ASR World for incidence was 83% higher in males than in females and 4% higher in peri-urban areas than in urban areas. The cumulative incidence rate for subjects aged 0 to 74 years was 1.27%（Table 5.5.5）.

表 5.5.5 2019 年北京市户籍居民直肠癌（C19-20）发病情况
Table 5.5.5 Incidence of rectal cancer （C19-20） in Beijing, 2019

地区 Area	性别 Sex	例数 No. of cases	粗率 Crude rate （1/10^5）	构成比 Freq.（%）	中标率 ASR China （1/10^5）	世标率 ASR World （1/10^5）	累积率 Cumulative rate（0~74, %）
全市 All areas	合计 Both	3 061	22.08	5.26	10.21	10.16	1.27
	男性 Male	1 940	28.14	6.79	13.21	13.27	1.66
	女性 Female	1 121	16.08	3.78	7.40	7.24	0.89
城区 Urban areas	合计 Both	1 933	22.63	5.08	10.07	10.03	1.28
	男性 Male	1 231	29.02	6.65	13.13	13.17	1.68
	女性 Female	702	16.32	3.59	7.18	7.03	0.89
郊区 Peri-urban areas	合计 Both	1 128	21.19	5.59	10.48	10.44	1.25
	男性 Male	709	26.73	7.04	13.42	13.53	1.62
	女性 Female	419	15.69	4.15	7.77	7.60	0.90

2019 年，北京市直肠癌（C19-20）死亡病例数为 1 311 例，占全部恶性肿瘤死亡的 4.79%；其中男性 807 例，女性 504 例，城区 853 例，郊区 458 例。直肠癌（C19-20）死亡率为 9.45/10 万，中标死亡率和世标死亡率均为 3.62/10 万；男性世标死亡率为女性的 1.79 倍，郊区世标死亡率为城区的 1.07 倍。0~74 岁累积死亡率为 0.36%（表 5.5.6）。

A total of 1,311 cases died of rectal cancer（C19-20; 807 males and 504 females, 853 in urban areas and 458 in peri-urban areas）, accounting for 4.79% of all cancer deaths in 2019. The crude mortality rate was 9.45 per 100,000, with both ASR China and ASR World of 3.62 per 100,000. The ASR World for mortality was 79% higher in males than in females and 7% higher in peri-urban areas than in urban areas. The cumulative mortality rate for subjects aged 0 to 74 years was 0.36%（Table 5.5.6）.

表 5.5.6 2019 年北京市户籍居民直肠癌（C19-20）死亡情况
Table 5.5.6 Mortality of rectal cancer （C19-20） in Beijing, 2019

地区 Area	性别 Sex	例数 No. of deaths	粗率 Crude rate （1/10⁵）	构成比 Freq.（%）	中标率 ASR China （1/10⁵）	世标率 ASR World （1/10⁵）	累积率 Cumulative rate（0~74, %）
全市 All areas	合计 Both	1 311	9.45	4.79	3.62	3.62	0.36
	男性 Male	807	11.70	4.98	4.73	4.72	0.49
	女性 Female	504	7.23	4.52	2.62	2.63	0.25
城区 Urban areas	合计 Both	853	9.98	4.78	3.55	3.56	0.37
	男性 Male	520	12.26	5.02	4.61	4.62	0.51
	女性 Female	333	7.74	4.45	2.59	2.59	0.25
郊区 Peri-urban areas	合计 Both	458	8.60	4.82	3.81	3.81	0.35
	男性 Male	287	10.82	4.92	5.06	5.03	0.45
	女性 Female	171	6.40	4.66	2.69	2.73	0.26

北京市结直肠癌世标发病率由2010年的17.14/10万上升到2019年的23.73/10万，年均变化百分比为3.00%（*P* < 0.001）；男性和女性世标发病率10年间年均变化百分比分别为3.83%（*P* < 0.001）和1.89%（*P*=0.001）。北京市结直肠癌世标死亡率2010年为8.11/10万，2019年为8.39/10万，年均变化百分比为0.51%（*P*=0.110）；男性和女性世标死亡率10年间年均变化百分比分别为1.30%（*P*=0.012）和-0.54%（*P*=0.150）。

结直肠癌年龄别发病率和死亡率在男性和女性中均随年龄增长呈上升趋势：年龄别发病率从40~44岁年龄组开始上升明显，至80~84岁年龄组达高峰；年龄别死亡率从40~44岁年龄组开始持续上升，至85岁及以上年龄组达高峰（图5.5.1至图5.5.6）。50岁以上年龄组男性各年龄别发病率和死亡率均明显高于女性（图5.5.1和图5.5.4）。城区和郊区年龄别发病率、死亡率变化有一定差异，但总体趋势相同（图5.5.2和图5.5.3，图5.5.5和图5.5.6）。

The ASR World for incidence of colorectal cancer increased from 17.14 per 100,000 in 2010 to 23.73 per 100,000 in 2019; and the APC of ASR World for incidence was 3.00%（*P* < 0.001）. The APCs of ASR World for incidence of colorectal cancer in males and females were 3.83%（*P* < 0.001）and 1.89%（*P*=0.001）, respectively. The ASR World for mortality of colorectal cancer was 8.11 per 100,000 in 2010 and 8.39 per 100,000 in 2019; and the APC of ASR World for mortality was 0.51%（*P*=0.110）. The APCs of ASR World for mortality of colorectal cancer in males and females were 1.30%（*P*=0.012）and -0.54%（*P*=0.150）, respectively.

Trends of age-specific incidence and mortality rates of colorectal cancer were similar for males and females: the incidence rates for both sexes increased rapidly, starting with the age group of 40-44 years, and peaked at the age group of 80-84 years. The mortality rates increased consistently, starting with the age group of 40-44 years, and peaked at the age group of 85 years and above（Figure 5.5.1-5.5.6）. Age-specific incidence and mortality rates were consistently higher in males than in females, starting from the age group of 50 years old（Figure 5.5.1, Figure 5.5.4）. There were some differences in age-specific incidence and mortality rates between urban and peri-urban areas, but the overall trends were same（Figure 5.5.2-5.5.3, Figure 5.5.5-5.5.6）.

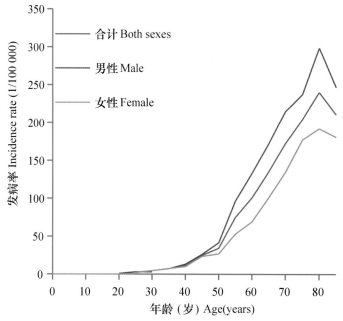

图5.5.1 2019年北京市户籍居民结直肠癌年龄别发病率

Figure 5.5.1 Age-specific incidence rates of colorectal cancer in Beijing, 2019

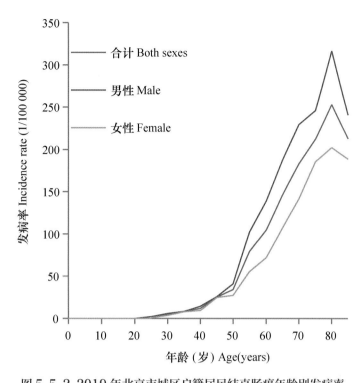

图 5.5.2 2019 年北京市城区户籍居民结直肠癌年龄别发病率
Figure 5.5.2 Age-specific incidence rates of colorectal cancer in urban areas of Beijing, 2019

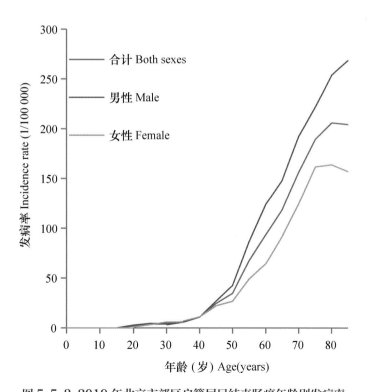

图 5.5.3 2019 年北京市郊区户籍居民结直肠癌年龄别发病率
Figure 5.5.3 Age-specific incidence rates of colorectal cancer in peri-urban areas of Beijing, 2019

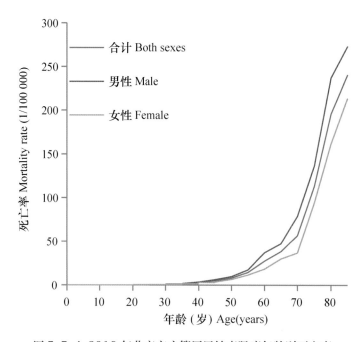

图 5.5.4 2019 年北京市户籍居民结直肠癌年龄别死亡率
Figure 5.5.4 Age-specific mortality rates of colorectal cancer in Beijing, 2019

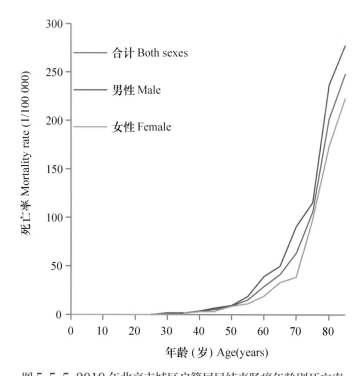

图 5.5.5 2019 年北京市城区户籍居民结直肠癌年龄别死亡率
Figure 5.5.5 Age-specific mortality rates of colorectal cancer in urban areas of Beijing, 2019

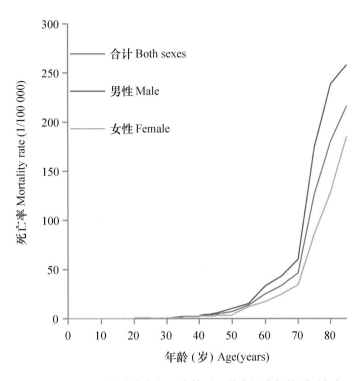

图 5.5.6 2019 年北京市郊区户籍居民结直肠癌年龄别死亡率
Figure 5.5.6 Age-specific mortality rates of colorectal cancer in peri-urban areas of Beijing, 2019

2019 年，北京市结直肠癌世标发病率和死亡率在 16 个辖区间存在一定差异，城区发病率和死亡率均高于郊区（图 5.5.7 和图 5.5.8）。

In 2019, there were some differences among the 16 districts in ASR World for incidence and mortality of colorectal cancer in Beijing. The incidence and mortality rates were both higher in urban areas than in peri-urban areas（Figure 5.5.7-5.5.8）.

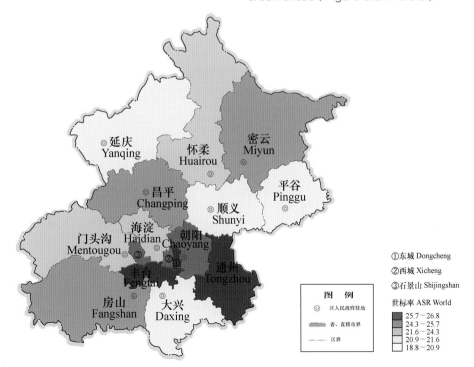

图 5.5.7 2019 年北京市户籍居民结直肠癌世标发病率（1/10⁵）地区分布情况
Figure 5.5.7 ASRs World for incidence of colorectal cancer（1/10⁵）by district in Beijing, 2019

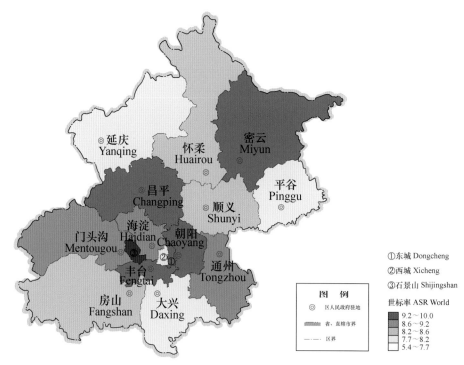

图 5.5.8 2019 年北京市户籍居民结直肠癌世标死亡率（1/10⁵）地区分布情况
Figure 5.5.8 ASRs World for mortality of colorectal cancer（1/10⁵）by district in Beijing, 2019

全部结肠癌（C18）新发病例中，有明确亚部位的病例占 79.25%。其中乙状结肠是最常见的发病部位，占 44.30%；其后依次为升结肠、降结肠和横结肠，分别占 23.63%、7.17% 和 7.02%（图 5.5.9）。

About 79.25% of new cases were assigned to specified categories of colon cancer（C18）site. Among those, the sigmoid colon was the most common site, accounting for 44.30% of all cases, followed by the ascending colon（23.63%）, the descending colon（7.17%）and the transverse colon（7.02%）(Figure 5.5.9).

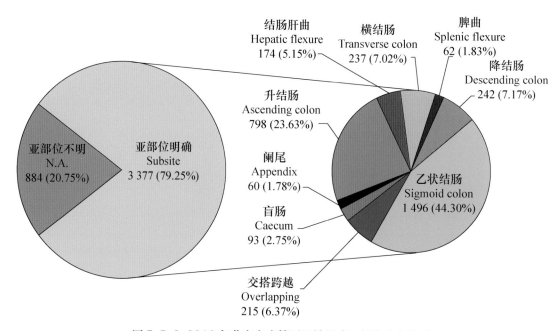

图 5.5.9 2019 年北京市户籍居民结肠癌亚部位分布情况
Figure 5.5.9 Subsite distribution of colon cancer in Beijing, 2019

（撰稿 张希，校稿 李浩鑫）

5.6 肝（C22）

2019年，北京市肝癌新发病例数为2 385例，占全部恶性肿瘤发病的4.10%，位居恶性肿瘤发病第6位；其中男性1 750例，女性635例，城区1 420例，郊区965例。肝癌发病率为17.20/10万，中标发病率为7.88/10万，世标发病率为7.93/10万；男性世标发病率为女性的3.44倍，郊区世标发病率为城区的1.29倍。0~74岁累积发病率为0.89%（表5.6.1）。

5.6 Liver（C22）

There were 2,385 new cases diagnosed as liver cancer（1,750 males and 635 females, 1,420 in urban areas and 965 in peri-urban areas）, accounting for 4.10% of new cases of all cancers in 2019. Liver cancer was the 6th common cancer in Beijing. The crude incidence rate was 17.20 per 100,000, with an ASR China and an ASR World of 7.88 and 7.93 per 100,000, respectively. The ASR World for incidence was 244% higher in males than in females and 29% higher in peri-urban areas than in urban areas. The cumulative incidence rate for subjects aged 0 to 74 years was 0.89%（Table 5.6.1）.

表 5.6.1 2019 年北京市户籍居民肝癌发病情况
Table 5.6.1 Incidence of liver cancer in Beijing, 2019

地区 Area	性别 Sex	例数 No. of cases	粗率 Crude rate （1/10^5）	构成比 Freq.（%）	中标率 ASR China （1/10^5）	世标率 ASR World （1/10^5）	累积率 Cumulative rate（0~74, %）	顺位 Rank
全市 All areas	合计 Both	2 385	17.20	4.10	7.88	7.93	0.89	6
	男性 Male	1 750	25.38	6.13	12.38	12.41	1.43	6
	女性 Female	635	9.11	2.14	3.53	3.60	0.38	12
城区 Urban areas	合计 Both	1 420	16.62	3.73	7.03	7.12	0.80	7
	男性 Male	1 042	24.56	5.63	11.18	11.26	1.31	6
	女性 Female	378	8.79	1.93	3.07	3.14	0.31	12
郊区 Peri-urban areas	合计 Both	965	18.13	4.79	9.20	9.19	1.04	5
	男性 Male	708	26.69	7.03	14.22	14.17	1.61	3
	女性 Female	257	9.62	2.55	4.31	4.37	0.48	8

2019年，北京市肝癌死亡病例数为1 966例，占全部恶性肿瘤死亡的7.19%，位居恶性肿瘤死亡第3位；其中男性1 424例，女性542例，城区1 165例，郊区801例。肝癌死亡率为14.18/10万，中标死亡率与世标死亡率均为6.10/10万；男性世标死亡率为女性的3.49倍，郊区世标死亡率为城区的1.35倍。0~74岁累积死亡率为0.69%（表5.6.2）。

A total of 1,966 cases died of liver cancer（1,424 males and 542 females, 1,165 in urban areas and 801 in peri-urban areas）, accounting for 7.19% of all cancer deaths in 2019. Liver cancer was the 3rd leading cause of cancer deaths in all cancers. The crude mortality rate was 14.18 per 100,000, with both ASR China and ASR World of 6.10 per 100,000. The ASR World for mortality was 249% higher in males than in females and 35% higher in peri-urban areas than in urban areas, respectively. The cumulative mortality rate for subjects aged 0 to 74 years was 0.69%（Table 5.6.2）.

表 5.6.2 2019 年北京市户籍居民肝癌死亡情况
Table 5.6.2 Mortality of liver cancer in Beijing, 2019

地区 Area	性别 Sex	例数 No. of deaths	粗率 Crude rate （1/10⁵）	构成比 Freq.（%）	中标率 ASR China （1/10⁵）	世标率 ASR World （1/10⁵）	累积率 Cumulative rate（0~74,%）	顺位 Rank
全市 All areas	合计 Both	1 966	14.18	7.19	6.10	6.10	0.69	3
	男性 Male	1 424	20.65	8.79	9.62	9.60	1.10	3
	女性 Female	542	7.77	4.86	2.75	2.75	0.29	6
城区 Urban areas	合计 Both	1 165	13.64	6.53	5.35	5.38	0.59	4
	男性 Male	840	19.80	8.10	8.49	8.51	0.97	4
	女性 Female	325	7.56	4.34	2.38	2.40	0.22	6
郊区 Peri-urban areas	合计 Both	801	15.05	8.43	7.29	7.24	0.84	3
	男性 Male	584	22.02	10.01	11.35	11.28	1.31	2
	女性 Female	217	8.13	5.92	3.40	3.37	0.38	4

北京市肝癌世标发病率由 2010 年的 11.77/10 万下降到 2019 年的 7.93/10 万，年均变化百分比为 -5.14%（$P < 0.001$）；男性和女性世标发病率 10 年间年均变化百分比分别为 -5.02%（$P < 0.001$）和 -5.44%（$P < 0.001$）。北京市肝癌世标死亡率由 2010 年的 9.76/10 万下降到 2019 年的 6.10/10 万，年均变化百分比为 -4.87%（$P < 0.001$）；男性和女性世标死亡率 10 年间年均变化百分比分别为 -4.63%（$P < 0.001$）和 -5.47%（$P < 0.001$）。

肝癌年龄别发病率和死亡率呈现明显的性别差异，除低年龄组略有波动外，30 岁以上各年龄组男性发病率与死亡率均高于女性。无论男女，肝癌年龄别发病率和死亡率 35 岁之前整体处于较低水平，35 岁之后开始快速升高，男性和女性的发病率和死亡率均在 85 岁及以上年龄组达到高峰。城区

The ASR World for incidence of liver cancer decreased from 11.77 per 100,000 in 2010 to 7.93 per 100,000 in 2019; and the APC of ASR World for incidence was -5.14% （$P < 0.001$）.The APCs of ASR World for incidence of liver cancer in males and females were -5.02% （$P < 0.001$）and -5.44% （$P < 0.001$）, respectively. The ASR World for mortality of liver cancer decreased from 9.76 per 100,000 in 2010 to 6.10 per 100,000 in 2019; and the APC of ASR World for mortality was -4.87% （$P < 0.001$）. The APCs of ASR World for mortality of liver cancer in males and females were -4.63%（$P < 0.001$）and -5.47%（$P < 0.001$）, respectively.

The trends of age-specific incidence and mortality rates showed differences between males and females in Beijing. Except for the slight fluctuation observed in lower age groups, age-specific incidence and mortality rates of liver cancer were consistently higher in males than in females starting from the age group of 30-34 years old. The age-specific incidence and mortality rates for both sexes were relatively low in people aged below 35 years old and increased sharply thereafter. The incidence and mortality rates for both males and females peaked at the age group of 85 years and

和郊区年龄别发病率、死亡率变化有一定差异（图 5.6.1 至图 5.6.6）。

above. There are some differences in age-specific incidence and mortality rates between urban and peri-urban areas（Figure 5.6.1-5.6.6）.

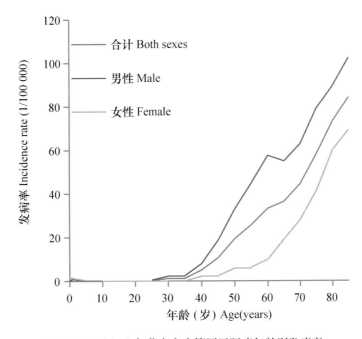

图 5.6.1 2019 年北京市户籍居民肝癌年龄别发病率
Figure 5.6.1 Age-specific incidence rates of liver cancer in Beijing, 2019

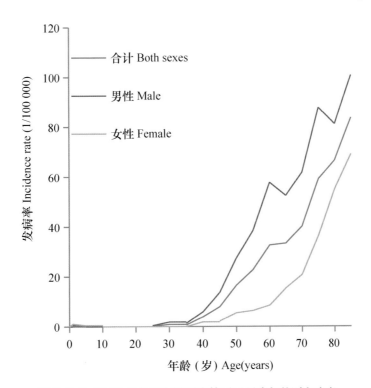

图 5.6.2 2019 年北京市城区户籍居民肝癌年龄别发病率
Figure 5.6.2 Age-specific incidence rates of liver cancer in urban areas of Beijing, 2019

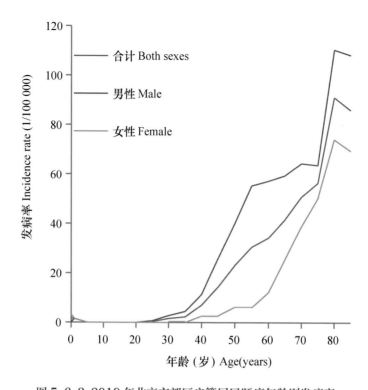

图 5.6.3 2019 年北京市郊区户籍居民肝癌年龄别发病率
Figure 5.6.3 Age-specific incidence rates of liver cancer in peri-urban areas of Beijing, 2019

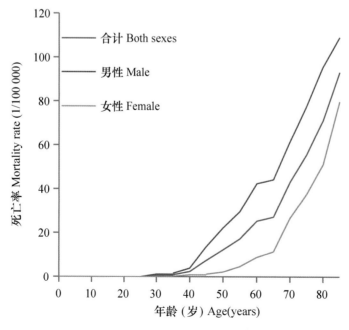

图 5.6.4 2019 年北京市户籍居民肝癌年龄别死亡率
Figure 5.6.4 Age-specific mortality rates of liver cancer in Beijing, 2019

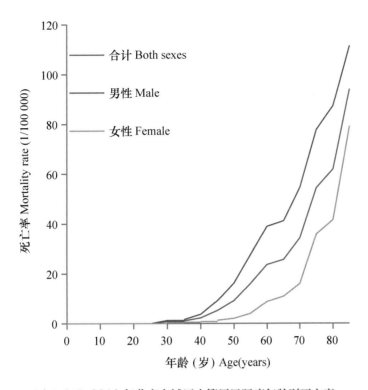

图 5.6.5 2019 年北京市城区户籍居民肝癌年龄别死亡率
Figure 5.6.5 Age-specific mortality rates of liver cancer in urban areas of Beijing, 2019

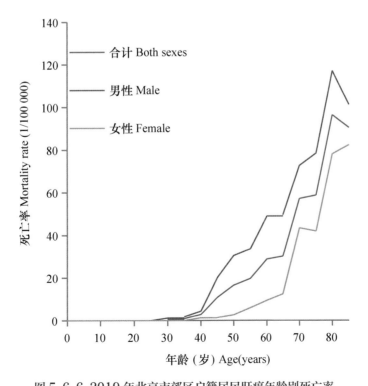

图 5.6.6 2019 年北京市郊区户籍居民肝癌年龄别死亡率
Figure 5.6.6 Age-specific mortality rates of liver cancer in peri-urban areas of Beijing, 2019

2019年，北京市肝癌世标发病率和死亡率在16个辖区间有一定差异，郊区发病率和死亡率均高于城区（图5.6.7和图5.6.8）。

In 2019, there were some differences among the 16 districts in ASR World for incidence and mortality of liver cancer in Beijing. The incidence and mortality rates were higher in peri-urban areas than in urban areas（Figure 5.6.7-5.6.8）.

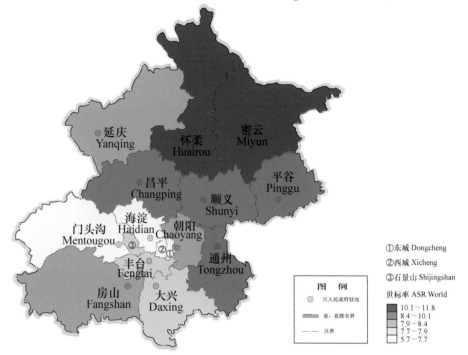

图 5.6.7 2019 年北京市户籍居民肝癌世标发病率（1/10⁵）地区分布情况
Figure 5.6.7 ASRs World for incidence of liver cancer（1/10⁵）by district in Beijing, 2019

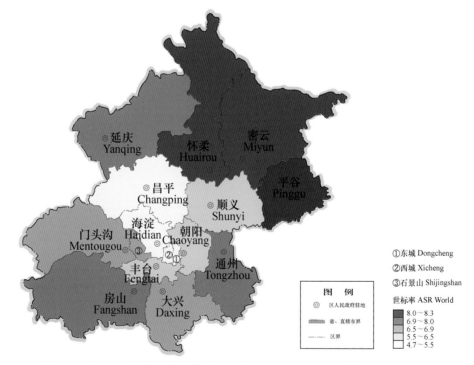

图 5.6.8 2019 年北京市户籍居民肝癌世标死亡率（1/10⁵）地区分布情况
Figure 5.6.8 ASRs World for mortality of liver cancer（1/10⁵）by district in Beijing, 2019

（撰稿 刘硕，校稿 李慧超）

5.7 胆囊（C23-24）

2019 年，北京市胆囊癌新发病例数为 1 240 例，占全部恶性肿瘤发病的 2.13%，位居恶性肿瘤发病第 14 位；其中男性 651 例，女性 589 例，城区 737 例，郊区 503 例。胆囊癌发病率为 8.94/10 万，中标发病率为 3.61/10 万，世标发病率为 3.59/10 万；男性世标发病率为女性的 1.30 倍，郊区世标发病率为城区的 1.35 倍。0~74 岁累积发病率为 0.40%（表 5.7.1）。

5.7 Gallbladder（C23-24）

There were 1,240 new cases diagnosed as gallbladder cancer（651 males and 589 females, 737 in urban areas and 503 in peri-urban areas）, accounting for 2.13% of new cases of all cancers in 2019. Gallbladder cancer was the 14th common cancer in Beijing. The crude incidence rate was 8.94 per 100,000, with an ASR China and an ASR World of 3.61 and 3.59 per 100,000, respectively. The ASR World for incidence was 30% higher in males than in females and 35% higher in peri-urban areas than in urban areas. The cumulative incidence rate for subjects aged 0 to 74 years was 0.40%（Table 5.7.1）.

表 5.7.1 2019 年北京市户籍居民胆囊癌发病情况
Table 5.7.1 Incidence of gallbladder cancer in Beijing, 2019

地区 Area	性别 Sex	例数 No. of cases	粗率 Crude rate （1/10^5）	构成比 Freq.（%）	中标率 ASR China （1/10^5）	世标率 ASR World （1/10^5）	累积率 Cumulative rate（0~74, %）	顺位 Rank
全市 All areas	合计 Both	1 240	8.94	2.13	3.61	3.59	0.40	14
	男性 Male	651	9.44	2.28	4.05	4.07	0.46	13
	女性 Female	589	8.45	1.99	3.19	3.14	0.35	13
城区 Urban areas	合计 Both	737	8.63	1.94	3.23	3.20	0.36	14
	男性 Male	361	8.51	1.95	3.36	3.34	0.36	13
	女性 Female	376	8.74	1.92	3.10	3.06	0.36	13
郊区 Peri-urban areas	合计 Both	503	9.45	2.49	4.31	4.30	0.47	12
	男性 Male	290	10.93	2.88	5.24	5.33	0.62	11
	女性 Female	213	7.98	2.11	3.43	3.34	0.33	14

2019 年，北京市胆囊癌死亡病例数为 1 034 例，占全部恶性肿瘤死亡的 3.78%，位居恶性肿瘤死亡第 7 位；其中男性 535 例，女性 499 例，城区 615 例，郊区 419 例。胆囊癌死亡率为 7.46/10 万，中标死亡率为 2.82/10 万，世标死亡率为 2.81/10 万；男性世标死亡率为女性的 1.29 倍，郊区世标死亡率为城区的 1.43 倍。0~74 岁累积死亡率为 0.31%（表 5.7.2）。

A total of 1,034 cases died of gallbladder cancer（535 males and 499 females, 615 in urban areas and 419 in peri-urban areas）, accounting for 3.78% of all cancer deaths in 2019. Gallbladder cancer was the 7th leading cause of cancer deaths in all cancers. The crude mortality rate was 7.46 per 100,000, with an ASR China and an ASR World of 2.82 and 2.81 per 100,000, respectively. The ASR World for mortality was 29% higher in males than in females and 43% higher in peri-urban areas than in urban areas. The cumulative mortality rate for subjects aged 0 to 74 years was 0.31%（Table 5.7.2）.

表 5.7.2 2019 年北京市户籍居民胆囊癌死亡情况
Table 5.7.2 Mortality of gallbladder cancer in Beijing, 2019

地区 Area	性别 Sex	例数 No. of deaths	粗率 Crude rate （1/10⁵）	构成比 Freq.（%）	中标率 ASR China （1/10⁵）	世标率 ASR World （1/10⁵）	累积率 Cumulative rate（0~74, %）	顺位 Rank
全市 All areas	合计 Both	1 034	7.46	3.78	2.82	2.81	0.31	7
	男性 Male	535	7.76	3.30	3.16	3.17	0.35	11
	女性 Female	499	7.16	4.48	2.49	2.46	0.27	7
城区 Urban areas	合计 Both	615	7.20	3.45	2.45	2.43	0.26	9
	男性 Male	314	7.40	3.03	2.72	2.71	0.28	12
	女性 Female	301	7.00	4.02	2.18	2.15	0.24	9
郊区 Peri-urban areas	合计 Both	419	7.87	4.41	3.47	3.48	0.40	7
	男性 Male	221	8.33	3.79	3.92	3.96	0.47	7
	女性 Female	198	7.41	5.40	3.04	3.02	0.33	5

北京市胆囊癌世标发病率2010年为3.69/10万，2019年为3.59/10万，年均变化百分比为－0.39%（$P=0.401$）；男性和女性世标发病率10年间年均变化百分比分别为0.87%（$P=0.081$）和－1.79%（$P=0.006$）。北京市胆囊癌世标死亡率2010年为2.79/10万，2019年为2.81/10万，年均变化百分比为－0.63%（$P=0.353$）；男性和女性世标死亡率10年间年均变化百分比分别为0.89%（$P=0.121$）和－2.26%（$P=0.061$）。

胆囊癌年龄别发病率和死亡率在40岁以前均较低，40岁以后快速上升（图5.7.1至图5.7.6）。除70~74岁年龄组女性死亡率高于男性外，40岁以上年龄组男性胆囊癌发病率和死亡率均高于女性。男性和女性的发病率和死亡率均在80~84岁年龄组达到高峰（图5.7.1和图5.7.4）。城区和郊区年龄别发病率、死亡率变化有一定差异，但总体趋势相同（图5.7.2和图5.7.3，图5.7.5和图5.7.6）。

The ASR World for incidence of gallbladder cancer was 3.69 per 100,000 in 2010 and 3.59 per 100,000 in 2019; and the APC of ASR World for incidence was －0.39%（$P=0.401$）. The APCs of ASR World for incidence of gallbladder cancer in males and females were 0.87%（$P=0.081$）and －1.79%（$P=0.006$）, respectively. The ASR World for mortality of gallbladder cancer was 2.79 per 100,000 in 2010 and 2.81 per 100,000 in 2019; and the APC of ASR World for mortality was －0.63%（$P=0.353$）. The APCs of ASR World for mortality of gallbladder cancer in males and females were 0.89%（$P=0.121$）and －2.26%（$P=0.061$）, respectively.

The age-specific incidence and mortality rates of gallbladder cancer were relatively low in people below 40 years old, and the rates increased sharply in people older than that（Figure 5.7.1-5.7.6）. Except the mortality rate at the age group of 70-74 years was higher in females than in males, the incidence and mortality rates in males were consistently higher than those in females after 40 years old. And the age-specific incidence and mortality rates for both sexes peaked at the age group of 80-84 years（Figure 5.7.1, Figure 5.7.4）. There were some differences in age-specific incidence and mortality rates between urban and peri-urban areas, but the overall trends were same（Figure 5.7.2-5.7.3, Figure 5.7.5-5.7.6）.

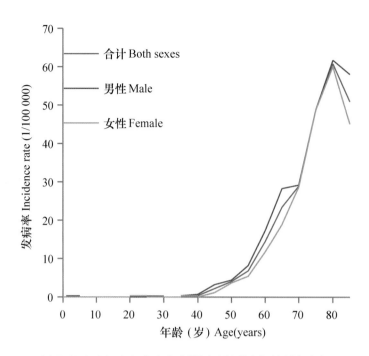

图 5.7.1 2019 年北京市户籍居民胆囊癌年龄别发病率
Figure 5.7.1 Age-specific incidence rates of gallbladder cancer in Beijing, 2019

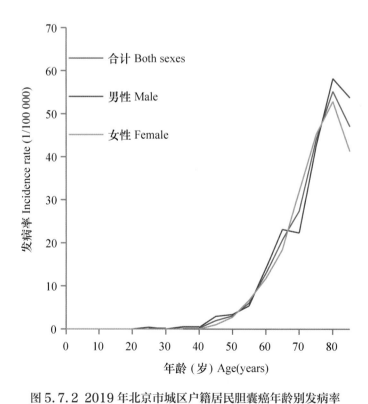

图 5.7.2 2019 年北京市城区户籍居民胆囊癌年龄别发病率
Figure 5.7.2 Age-specific incidence rates of gallbladder cancer in urban areas of Beijing, 2019

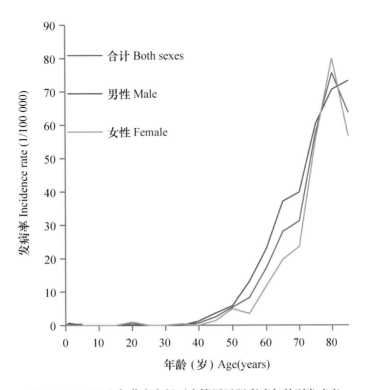

图 5.7.3 2019 年北京市郊区户籍居民胆囊癌年龄别发病率
Figure 5.7.3 Age-specific incidence rates of gallbladder cancer in peri-urban areas of Beijing, 2019

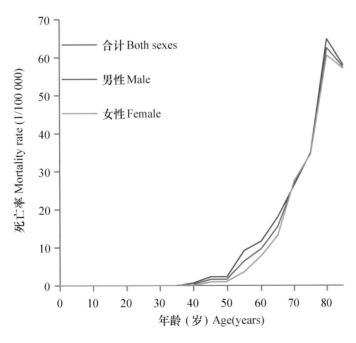

图 5.7.4 2019 年北京市户籍居民胆囊癌年龄别死亡率
Figure 5.7.4 Age-specific mortality rates of gallbladder cancer in Beijing, 2019

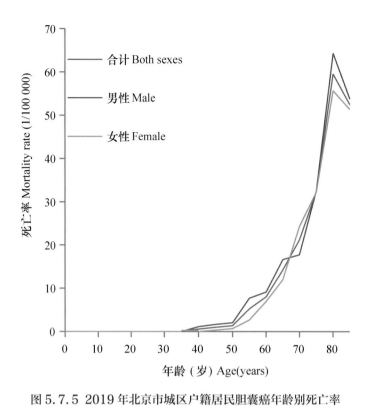

图 5.7.5 2019 年北京市城区户籍居民胆囊癌年龄别死亡率
Figure 5.7.5 Age-specific mortality rates of gallbladder cancer in urban areas of Beijing, 2019

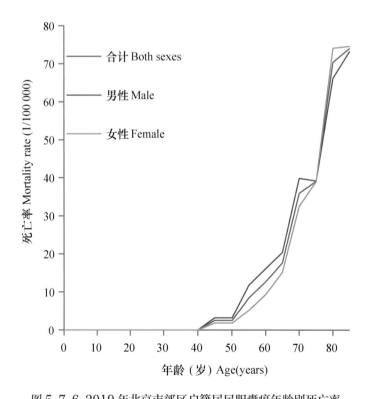

图 5.7.6 2019 年北京市郊区户籍居民胆囊癌年龄别死亡率
Figure 5.7.6 Age-specific mortality rates of gallbladder cancer in peri-urban areas of Beijing, 2019

（撰稿 刘硕，校稿 李慧超）

5.8 胰腺（C25）

2019 年，北京市胰腺癌新发病例数为 1 575 例，占全部恶性肿瘤发病的 2.70%，位居恶性肿瘤发病第 11 位；其中男性 802 例，女性 773 例，城区 1 093 例，郊区 482 例。胰腺癌发病率为 11.36/10 万，中标发病率为 4.76/10 万，世标发病率为 4.75/10 万；男性世标发病率为女性的 1.24 倍，城区世标发病率为郊区的 1.17 倍。0~74 岁累积发病率为 0.55%（表 5.8.1）。

5.8 Pancreas（C25）

There were 1,575 new cases diagnosed as pancreatic cancer（802 males and 773 females, 1,093 in urban areas and 482 in peri-urban areas）, accounting for 2.70% of new cases of all cancers in 2019. Pancreatic cancer was the 11th common cancer in Beijing. The crude incidence rate was 11.36 per 100,000, with an ASR China and an ASR World of 4.76 and 4.75 per 100,000, respectively. The ASR World for incidence was 24% higher in males than in females and 17% higher in urban areas than in peri-urban areas. The cumulative incidence rate for subjects aged 0 to 74 years was 0.55%（Table 5.8.1）.

表 5.8.1 2019 年北京市户籍居民胰腺癌发病情况
Table 5.8.1 Incidence of pancreatic cancer in Beijing, 2019

地区 Area	性别 Sex	例数 No. of cases	粗率 Crude rate （1/10⁵）	构成比 Freq.（%）	中标率 ASR China （1/10⁵）	世标率 ASR World （1/10⁵）	累积率 Cumulative rate（0~74, %）	顺位 Rank
全市 All areas	合计 Both	1 575	11.36	2.70	4.76	4.75	0.55	11
	男性 Male	802	11.63	2.81	5.24	5.26	0.63	11
	女性 Female	773	11.09	2.61	4.28	4.24	0.46	9
城区 Urban areas	合计 Both	1 093	12.79	2.87	5.04	5.02	0.58	11
	男性 Male	545	12.85	2.95	5.48	5.51	0.67	10
	女性 Female	548	12.74	2.80	4.58	4.52	0.50	9
郊区 Peri-urban areas	合计 Both	482	9.06	2.39	4.29	4.28	0.49	14
	男性 Male	257	9.69	2.55	4.85	4.85	0.58	13
	女性 Female	225	8.43	2.23	3.74	3.73	0.41	14

2019 年，北京市胰腺癌死亡病例数为 1 445 例，占全部恶性肿瘤死亡的 5.28%，位居恶性肿瘤死亡第 5 位；其中男性 739 例，女性 706 例，城区 1 014 例，郊区 431 例。胰腺癌死亡率为 10.42/10 万，中标死亡率为 4.16/10 万，世标死亡率为 4.15/10 万；男性世标死亡率为女性的 1.30 倍，城区世标死亡率为郊区的 1.20 倍。0~74 岁累积死亡率为 0.46%（表 5.8.2）。

A total of 1,445 cases died of pancreatic cancer（739 males and 706 females, 1,014 in urban areas and 431 in peri-urban areas）, accounting for 5.28% of all cancer deaths in 2019. Pancreatic cancer was the 5th leading cause of cancer deaths in all cancers. The crude mortality rate was 10.42 per 100,000, with an ASR China and an ASR World of 4.16 and 4.15 per 100,000, respectively. The ASR World for mortality was 30% higher in males than in females and 20% higher in urban areas than in peri-urban areas. The cumulative mortality rate for subjects aged 0 to 74 years was 0.46%（Table 5.8.2）.

表 5.8.2 2019 年北京市户籍居民胰腺癌死亡情况
Table 5.8.2 Mortality of pancreatic cancer in Beijing, 2019

地区 Area	性别 Sex	例数 No. of deaths	粗率 Crude rate （1/10⁵）	构成比 Freq.（%）	中标率 ASR China （1/10⁵）	世标率 ASR World （1/10⁵）	累积率 Cumulative rate（0~74, %）	顺位 Rank
全市 All areas	合计 Both	1 445	10.42	5.28	4.16	4.15	0.46	5
	男性 Male	739	10.72	4.56	4.67	4.69	0.55	6
	女性 Female	706	10.13	6.33	3.65	3.61	0.37	4
城区 Urban areas	合计 Both	1 014	11.87	5.68	4.40	4.40	0.49	5
	男性 Male	502	11.83	4.84	4.83	4.89	0.58	6
	女性 Female	512	11.90	6.84	3.95	3.91	0.40	4
郊区 Peri-urban areas	合计 Both	431	8.10	4.54	3.73	3.67	0.40	6
	男性 Male	237	8.93	4.06	4.42	4.34	0.49	6
	女性 Female	194	7.27	5.29	3.09	3.05	0.32	6

北京市胰腺癌世标发病率 2010 年为 4.60/10 万，2019 年为 4.75/10 万，年均变化百分比为 -0.17%（P=0.490）；男性和女性世标发病率 10 年间年均变化百分比分别为 0.03%（P=0.953）和 -0.46%（P=0.523）。北京市胰

The ASR World for incidence of pancreatic cancer was 4.60 per 100,000 in 2010 and 4.75 per 100,000 in 2019; and the APC of ASR World for incidence was -0.17%（P=0.490）. The APCs of ASR World for incidence of pancreatic cancer in males and females were 0.03%（P=0.953）and -0.46%（P=0.523）, respectively. The ASR World for mortality of pancreatic cancer was 4.22 per 100,000 in 2010 and

腺癌世标死亡率 2010 年为 4.22/10 万，2019 年为 4.15/10 万，年均变化百分比为 − 0.16%（$P = 0.468$）；男性和女性世标死亡率 10 年间年均变化百分比分别为 0.20%（$P = 0.704$）和 − 0.71%（$P = 0.335$）。

　　胰腺癌年龄别发病率和死亡率在 45 岁以前均较低，45 岁以后快速上升，在 85 岁及以上年龄组达到高峰（图 5.8.1 至图 5.8.6）。除 75 ~ 79 岁、80 ~ 84 岁和 85 岁及以上年龄组女性发病率和死亡率高于男性外，45 岁以上年龄组男性胰腺癌发病率和死亡率均高于女性。男性的发病率与死亡率均在 85 岁及以上年龄组达到高峰，而女性的发病率与死亡率均在 80 ~ 84 岁年龄组达到高峰（图 5.8.1 和图 5.8.4）。城区和郊区年龄别发病率、死亡率变化存在差异，但总体趋势相同（图 5.8.2 和图 5.8.3，图 5.8.5 和图 5.8.6）。

4.15 per 100,000 in 2019; and the APC of ASR World for mortality was − 0.16%（$P = 0.468$）. The APCs of ASR World for mortality of pancreatic cancer in males and females were 0.20%（$P = 0.704$）and − 0.71%（$P = 0.335$）, respectively.

The age-specific incidence and mortality rates of pancreatic cancer were relatively low in people below 45 years old, and the rates increased sharply in people older than that. Furthermore, both the incidence and mortality rates peaked at the age group of 85 years and above（Figure 5.8.1-5.8.6）. Except for the incidence and mortality rates at the age group of 75 ~ 79 years, 80 ~ 84 years and 85 years and above were higher in females than in males, the incidence and mortality rates in males were consistently higher than those in females after 45 years old. The age-specific incidence and mortality rates for males both peaked at the age group of 85 years and above. And the age-specific incidence and mortality rates for females both peaked at the age group of 80-84 years（Figure 5.8.1, Figure 5.8.4）. There were some differences in age-specific incidence and mortality rates between urban and peri-urban areas, but the overall trends were same（Figure 5.8.2-5.8.3, Figure 5.8.5-5.8.6）.

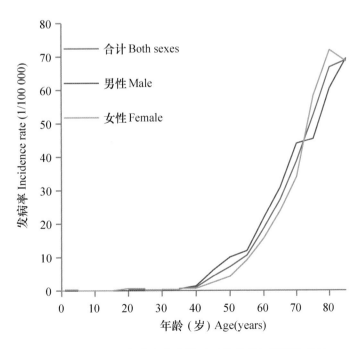

图 5.8.1　2019 年北京市户籍居民胰腺癌年龄别发病率
Figure 5.8.1　Age-specific incidence rates of pancreatic cancer in Beijing, 2019

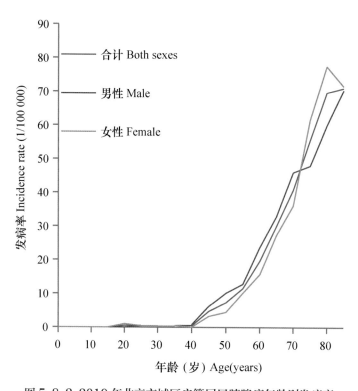

图 5.8.2 2019 年北京市城区户籍居民胰腺癌年龄别发病率
Figure 5.8.2 Age-specific incidence rates of pancreatic cancer in urban areas of Beijing, 2019

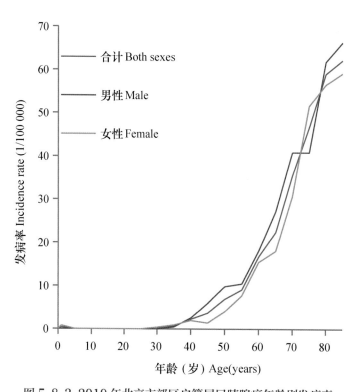

图 5.8.3 2019 年北京市郊区户籍居民胰腺癌年龄别发病率
Figure 5.8.3 Age-specific incidence rates of pancreatic cancer in peri-urban areas of Beijing, 2019

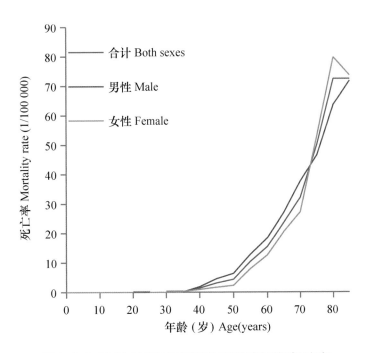

图 5.8.4 2019 年北京市户籍居民胰腺癌年龄别死亡率
Figure 5.8.4 Age-specific mortality rates of pancreatic cancer in Beijing, 2019

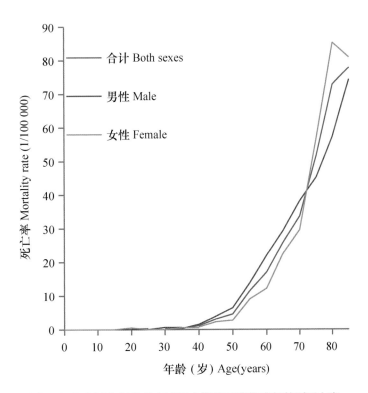

图 5.8.5 2019 年北京市城区户籍居民胰腺癌年龄别死亡率
Figure 5.8.5 Age-specific mortality rates of pancreatic cancer in urban areas of Beijing, 2019

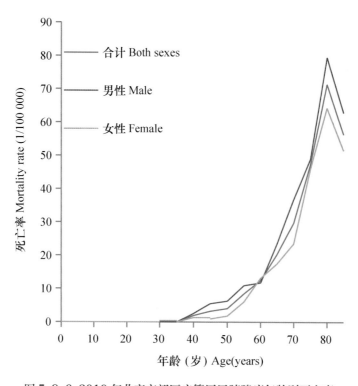

图 5.8.6 2019 年北京市郊区户籍居民胰腺癌年龄别死亡率
Figure 5.8.6 Age-specific mortality rates of pancreatic cancer in peri-urban areas of Beijing, 2019

全部胰腺癌新发病例中，有明确亚部位的病例占 27.11%。其中胰头是最常见的发病部位，占 67.92%；其后依次为胰尾、胰体和胰其他部位，分别占 12.41%、12.18% 和 3.28%（图 5.8.7）。

About 27.11% of new cases were assigned to specified categories of pancreatic cancer site. Among those, the head of pancreas was the most common subsite, accounting for 67.92% of all cases, followed by the tail (12.41%), the body (12.18%) and the other parts (3.28%)(Figure 5.8.7).

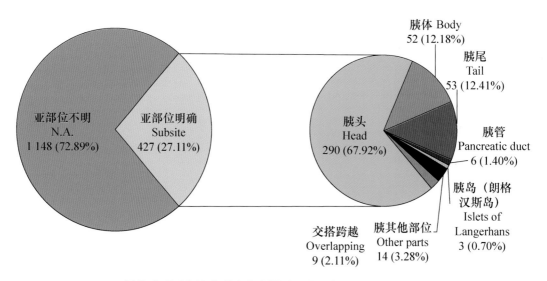

图 5.8.7 2019 年北京市户籍居民胰腺癌亚部位分布情况
Figure 5.8.7 Subsite distribution of pancreatic cancer in Beijing, 2019

（撰稿 李浩鑫，校稿 张希）

5.9 喉（C32）

2019 年，北京市喉癌新发病例数为 319 例，占全部恶性肿瘤发病的 0.55%，位居恶性肿瘤发病第 20 位；其中男性 302 例，女性 17 例，城区 186 例，郊区 133 例。喉癌发病率为 2.30/10 万，中标发病率为 1.05/10 万，世标发病率为 1.07/10 万；男性世标发病率为女性的 21.80 倍，郊区世标发病率为城区的 1.29 倍。0~74 岁累积发病率为 0.13%（表 5.9.1）。

5.9 Larynx（C32）

There were 319 new cases diagnosed as larynx cancer（302 males and 17 females, 186 in urban areas and 133 in peri-urban areas）, accounting for 0.55% of new cases of all cancers in 2019. Larynx cancer was the 20th common cancer in Beijing. The crude incidence rate was 2.30 per 100,000, with an ASR China and an ASR World of 1.05 and 1.07 per 100,000, respectively. The ASR World for incidence was 2 080% higher in males than in females and 29% higher in peri-urban areas than in urban areas. The cumulative incidence rate for subjects aged 0 to 74 years was 0.13%（Table 5.9.1）.

表 5.9.1 2019 年北京市户籍居民喉癌发病情况
Table 5.9.1 Incidence of larynx cancer in Beijing, 2019

地区 Area	性别 Sex	例数 No. of cases	粗率 Crude rate （1/10⁵）	构成比 Freq.（%）	中标率 ASR China （1/10⁵）	世标率 ASR World （1/10⁵）	累积率 Cumulative rate（0~74, %）	顺位 Rank
全市 All areas	合计 Both	319	2.30	0.55	1.05	1.07	0.13	20
	男性 Male	302	4.38	1.06	2.04	2.10	0.26	16
	女性 Female	17	0.24	0.06	0.10	0.10	0.01	23
城区 Urban areas	合计 Both	186	2.18	0.49	0.95	0.97	0.12	20
	男性 Male	176	4.15	0.95	1.84	1.89	0.24	16
	女性 Female	10	0.23	0.05	0.10	0.09	0.01	23
郊区 Peri-urban areas	合计 Both	133	2.50	0.66	1.21	1.25	0.15	20
	男性 Male	126	4.75	1.25	2.38	2.46	0.30	16
	女性 Female	7	0.26	0.07	0.10	0.11	0.01	23

2019年，北京市喉癌死亡病例数为144例，占全部恶性肿瘤死亡的0.53%，位居恶性肿瘤死亡第19位；其中男性138例，女性6例，城区83例，郊区61例。喉癌死亡率为1.04/10万，中标死亡率为0.38/10万，世标死亡率为0.39/10万；男性世标死亡率为女性的36.46倍，郊区世标死亡率为城区的1.41倍。0~74岁累积死亡率为0.04%（表5.9.2）。

A total of 144 cases died of larynx cancer（138 males and 6 females, 83 in urban areas and 61 in peri-urban areas）, accounting for 0.53% of all cancer deaths in 2019. Larynx cancer was the 19th leading cause of cancer deaths in all cancers. The crude mortality rate was 1.04 per 100,000, with an ASR China and an ASR World of 0.38 and 0.39 per 100,000, respectively. The ASR World for mortality was 3 546% higher in males than in females and 41% higher in peri-urban areas than in urban areas, respectively. The cumulative mortality rate for subjects aged 0 to 74 years was 0.04%（Table 5.9.2）.

表 5.9.2 2019 年北京市户籍居民喉癌死亡情况
Table 5.9.2 Mortality of larynx cancer in Beijing, 2019

地区 Area	性别 Sex	例数 No. of deaths	粗率 Crude rate （1/10⁵）	构成比 Freq.（%）	中标率 ASR China （1/10⁵）	世标率 ASR World （1/10⁵）	累积率 Cumulative rate（0~74, %）	顺位 Rank
全市 All areas	合计 Both	144	1.04	0.53	0.38	0.39	0.04	19
	男性 Male	138	2.00	0.85	0.78	0.80	0.09	15
	女性 Female	6	0.09	0.05	0.02	0.02	0.00	23
城区 Urban areas	合计 Both	83	0.97	0.47	0.33	0.35	0.04	19
	男性 Male	80	1.89	0.77	0.67	0.70	0.08	15
	女性 Female	3	0.07	0.04	0.02	0.02	0.00	23
郊区 Peri-urban areas	合计 Both	61	1.15	0.64	0.49	0.49	0.05	19
	男性 Male	58	2.19	0.99	1.00	1.00	0.10	15
	女性 Female	3	0.11	0.08	0.03	0.03	0.00	23

北京市喉癌世标发病率 2010 年为 1.15/10 万，2019 年为 1.07/10 万，年均变化百分比为 −0.74%（P=0.070）；男性和女性世标发病率 10 年间年均变化百分比分别为 −0.15%（P=0.728）和 −8.83%（P=0.001）。北京市喉癌世标死亡率 2010 年为 0.40/10 万，2019 年为 0.39/10 万，年均变化百分比为 −1.16%（P=0.388）；男性和女性世标死亡率 10 年间年均变化百分比分别为 0.24%（P=0.838）和 −13.36%（P=0.011）。

喉癌年龄别发病率在 35 岁以前均为 0，45 岁以后快速上升；年龄别死亡率在 40 岁以前均为 0，50 岁以后快速上升（图 5.9.1 至图 5.9.6）。男性喉癌年龄别发病率、死亡率及其上升速度均高于女性。男性和女性发病率均在 75~79 岁年龄组达到高峰，死亡率均在 85 岁及以上年龄组达到高峰（图 5.9.1 和图 5.9.4）。城区和郊区年龄别发病率、死亡率变化有一定差异，但总体趋势相同（图 5.9.2 和图 5.9.3，图 5.9.5 和图 5.9.6）。

The ASR World for incidence of larynx cancer was 1.15 per 100,000 in 2010 and 1.07 per 100,000 in 2019; and the APC of ASR World for incidence was −0.74%（P=0.070）. The APCs of ASR World for incidence of larynx cancer in males and females were −0.15%（P=0.728）and −8.83%（P=0.001）, respectively. The ASR World for mortality of larynx cancer was 0.40 per 100,000 in 2010 and 0.39 per 100,000 in 2019; and the APC of ASR World for mortality was −1.16%（P=0.388）. The APCs of ASR World for mortality of larynx cancer in males and females were 0.24%（P=0.838）and −13.36%（P=0.011）, respectively.

The age-specific incidence rates of larynx cancer were zero in people below 35 years old, and increased sharply in people older than 45 years old; the age-specific mortality rates of larynx cancer were zero in people below 40 years old, and increased sharply in people older than 50 years old（Figure 5.9.1-5.9.6）. The age-specific incidence and mortality rates and their growth rates in males were consistently higher than those in females across all age groups. The age-specific incidence rates for both sexes peaked at the age group of 75-79 years, while the age-specific mortality rates for both sexes peaked at the age group of 85 years and above（Figure 5.9.1, Figure 5.9.4）. There were some differences in age-specific incidence and mortality rates between urban and peri-urban areas, but the overall trends were same（Figure 5.9.2-5.9.3, Figure 5.9.5-5.9.6）.

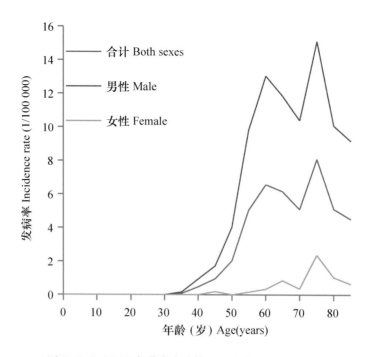

图 5.9.1 2019 年北京市户籍居民喉癌年龄别发病率
Figure 5.9.1 Age-specific incidence rates of larynx cancer in Beijing, 2019

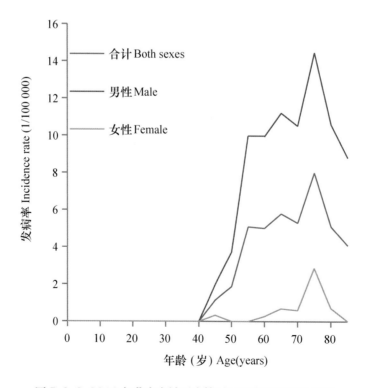

图 5.9.2 2019 年北京市城区户籍居民喉癌年龄别发病率
Figure 5.9.2 Age-specific incidence rates of larynx cancer in urban areas of Beijing, 2019

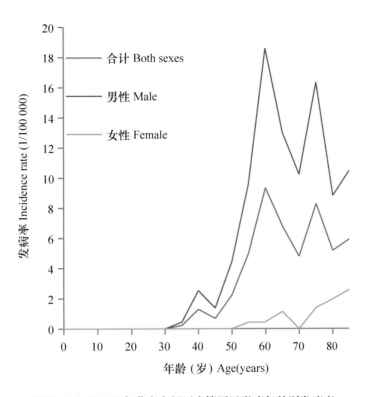

图 5.9.3 2019 年北京市郊区户籍居民喉癌年龄别发病率

Figure 5.9.3 Age-specific incidence rates of larynx cancer in peri-urban areas of Beijing, 2019

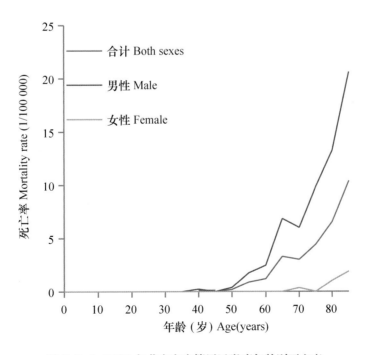

图 5.9.4 2019 年北京市户籍居民喉癌年龄别死亡率

Figure 5.9.4 Age-specific mortality rates of larynx cancer in Beijing, 2019

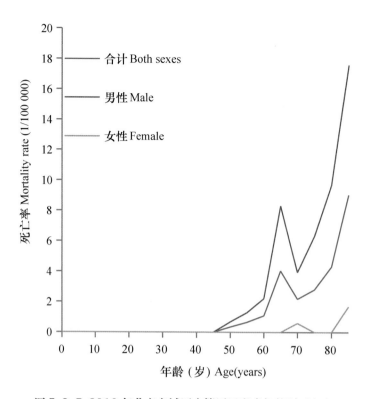

图 5.9.5 2019 年北京市城区户籍居民喉癌年龄别死亡率
Figure 5.9.5 Age-specific mortality rates of larynx cancer in urban areas of Beijing, 2019

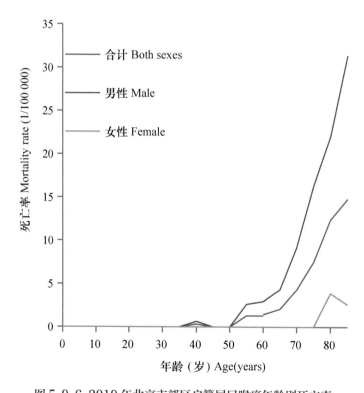

图 5.9.6 2019 年北京市郊区户籍居民喉癌年龄别死亡率
Figure 5.9.6 Age-specific mortality rates of larynx cancer in peri-urban areas of Beijing, 2019

（撰稿 李晴雨，校稿 刘硕）

5.10 肺（C33-34）

　　2019 年，北京市肺癌新发病例数为 12 646 例，占全部恶性肿瘤发病的 21.72%，位居恶性肿瘤发病第 1 位；其中男性 7 148 例，女性 5 498 例，城区 7 982 例，郊区 4 664 例。肺癌发病率为 91.20/10 万，中标发病率为 41.28/10 万，世标发病率为 40.93/10 万；男性世标发病率为女性的 1.32 倍，郊区世标发病率为城区的 1.03 倍。0~74 岁累积发病率为 4.95%（表 5.10.1）。

5.10 Lung（C33-34）

There were 12,646 new cases diagnosed as lung cancer（7,148 males and 5,498 females, 7,982 in urban areas and 4,664 in peri-urban areas）, accounting for 21.72% of new cases of all cancers in 2019. Lung cancer was the most common cancer in Beijing. The crude incidence rate was 91.20 per 100,000, with an ASR China and an ASR World of 41.28 and 40.93 per 100,000, respectively. The ASR World for incidence was 32% higher in males than in females and 3% higher in peri-urban areas than in urban areas. The cumulative incidence rate for subjects aged 0 to 74 years was 4.95%（Table 5.10.1）.

表 5.10.1 2019 年北京市户籍居民肺癌发病情况
Table 5.10.1 Incidence of lung cancer in Beijing, 2019

地区 Area	性别 Sex	例数 No. of cases	粗率 Crude rate （1/10^5）	构成比 Freq.（%）	中标率 ASR China （1/10^5）	世标率 ASR World （1/10^5）	累积率 Cumulative rate（0~74, %）	顺位 Rank
全市 All areas	合计 Both	12 646	91.20	21.72	41.28	40.93	4.95	1
	男性 Male	7 148	103.68	25.02	47.00	47.01	5.86	1
	女性 Female	5 498	78.86	18.53	36.38	35.64	4.13	2
城区 Urban areas	合计 Both	7 982	93.43	20.97	41.03	40.62	4.92	1
	男性 Male	4 403	103.80	23.80	45.01	45.03	5.64	1
	女性 Female	3 579	83.21	18.29	37.79	36.90	4.27	2
郊区 Peri-urban areas	合计 Both	4 664	87.62	23.13	42.10	41.87	5.01	1
	男性 Male	2 745	103.48	27.25	50.71	50.76	6.20	1
	女性 Female	1 919	71.86	19.02	34.50	33.98	3.93	1

2019 年，北京市肺癌死亡病例数为 7 810 例，占全部恶性肿瘤死亡的 28.56%，位居恶性肿瘤死亡第 1 位；其中男性 5 112 例，女性 2 698 例，城区 4 765 例，郊区 3 045 例。肺癌死亡率为 56.32/10 万，中标死亡率为 21.63/10 万，世标死亡率为 21.46/10 万；男性世标死亡率为女性的 2.34 倍，郊区世标死亡率为城区的 1.31 倍。0 ~ 74 岁累积死亡率为 2.31%（表 5.10.2）。

A total of 7,810 cases died of lung cancer（5,112 males and 2,698 females, 4,765 in urban areas and 3,045 in peri-urban areas）, accounting for 28.56% of all cancer deaths in 2019, ranking the 1st among all cancers. The crude mortality rate was 56.32 per 100,000, with an ASR China and an ASR World of 21.63 and 21.46 per 100,000, respectively. The ASR World for mortality was 134% higher in males than in females and 31% higher in peri-urban areas than in urban areas, respectively. The cumulative mortality rate for subjects aged 0 to 74 years was 2.31%（Table 5.10.2）.

表 5.10.2 2019 年北京市户籍居民肺癌死亡情况
Table 5.10.2 Mortality of lung cancer in Beijing, 2019

地区 Area	性别 Sex	例数 No. of deaths	粗率 Crude rate （1/10^5）	构成比 Freq.（%）	中标率 ASR China （1/10^5）	世标率 ASR World （1/10^5）	累积率 Cumulative rate（0~74, %）	顺位 Rank
全市 All areas	合计 Both	7 810	56.32	28.56	21.63	21.46	2.31	1
	男性 Male	5 112	74.15	31.55	30.78	30.64	3.48	1
	女性 Female	2 698	38.70	24.20	13.35	13.09	1.23	1
城区 Urban areas	合计 Both	4 765	55.78	26.70	19.44	19.31	2.04	1
	男性 Male	3 088	72.80	29.79	27.86	27.79	3.12	1
	女性 Female	1 677	38.99	22.42	11.79	11.54	1.03	1
郊区 Peri-urban areas	合计 Both	3 045	57.20	32.05	25.52	25.26	2.74	1
	男性 Male	2 024	76.30	34.68	36.06	35.84	4.05	1
	女性 Female	1 021	38.24	27.85	16.02	15.73	1.54	1

北京市肺癌世标发病率由 2010 年的 32.61/10 万上升到 2019 年的 40.93/10 万，年均变化百分比为 1.73%（*P*=0.037）。男性和女性世标发病率 10 年间年均变化百分比分别为 0.62%（*P*=0.241）和 3.48%（*P*=0.009）。北京市肺癌世标死亡率由 2010 年的 25.58/10 万下降到 2019 年的 21.46/10 万，年均变化百分比为 −1.90%（*P* < 0.001）；男性和女性世标死亡率 10 年间年均变化百分比分别为 −0.99%（*P*=0.001）和 −3.50%（*P* < 0.001）。

肺癌年龄别发病率在 40 岁以前较低，40 岁以后快速上升，男性上升速度高于女性；年龄别死亡率在 45 岁以前均较低，45 岁以后快速上升（图 5.10.1 至图 5.10.6）。男性和女性的发病率分别在 75~79 岁组和 80~84 岁组达到高峰，死亡率均在 85 岁及以上年龄组达到高峰（图 5.10.1 和图 5.10.4）。城区和郊区年龄别发病率、死亡率变化有一定差异，但总体趋势相同（图 5.10.2 和图 5.10.3，图 5.10.5 和图 5.10.6）。

The ASR World for incidence of lung cancer increased from 32.61 per 100,000 in 2010 to 40.93 per 100,000 in 2019; and the APC of ASR World for incidence was 1.73%（*P*=0.037）. The APCs of ASR World for incidence of lung cancer in males and females were 0.62%（*P*=0.241）and 3.48%（*P*=0.009）, respectively. The ASR World for mortality of lung cancer decreased from 25.58 per 100,000 in 2010 to 21.46 per 100,000 in 2019; and the APC of ASR World for mortality was −1.90%（*P* < 0.001）. The APCs of ASR World for mortality of lung cancer in males and females were −0.99%（*P*=0.001）and −3.50%（*P* < 0.001）, respectively.

The age-specific incidence rates of lung cancer were relatively low in people below 40 years old and increased sharply in people older than that; the rates grew faster in males than in females with the advancing of age. The age-specific mortality rates were relatively low at the age groups below 45 years, while the rates increased sharply above 45 years old（Figure 5.10.1-5.10.6）. The age-specific incidence rates for males and females peaked at the age group of 75-79 years and 80-84 years, respectively; while the mortality rates peaked at the age group of 85 years and above for both sexes（Figure 5.10.1, Figure 5.10.4）. There were some differences in age-specific incidence and mortality rates between urban and peri-urban areas, but the overall trends were same（Figure 5.10.2-5.10.3, Figure 5.10.5-5.10.6）.

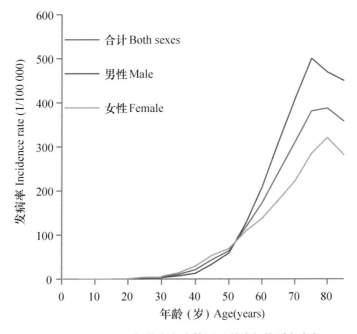

图 5.10.1 2019 年北京市户籍居民肺癌年龄别发病率
Figure 5.10.1 Age-specific incidence rates of lung cancer in Beijing, 2019

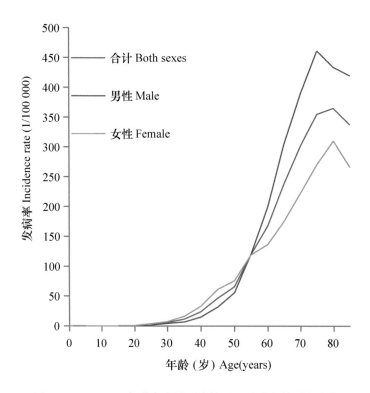

图 5.10.2 2019 年北京市城区户籍居民肺癌年龄别发病率
Figure 5.10.2 Age-specific incidence rates of lung cancer in urban areas of Beijing, 2019

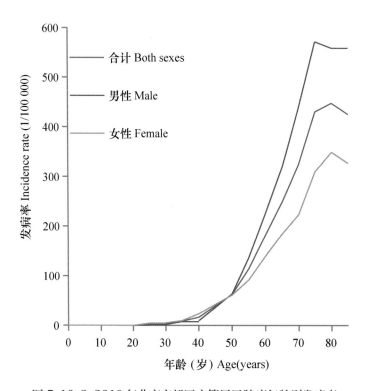

图 5.10.3 2019 年北京市郊区户籍居民肺癌年龄别发病率
Figure 5.10.3 Age-specific incidence rates of lung cancer in peri-urban areas of Beijing, 2019

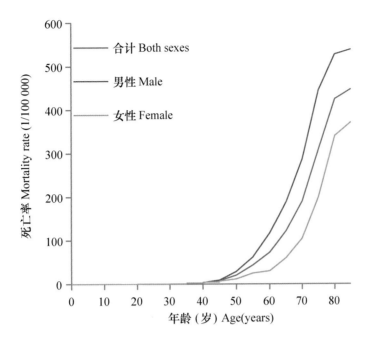

图 5.10.4 2019 年北京市户籍居民肺癌年龄别死亡率
Figure 5.10.4 Age-specific mortality rates of lung cancer in Beijing, 2019

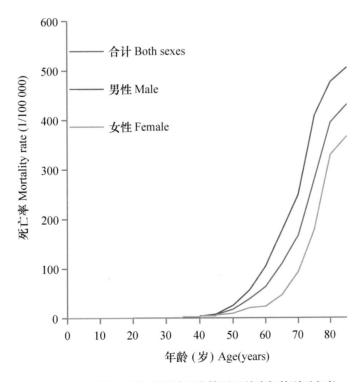

图 5.10.5 2019 年北京市城区户籍居民肺癌年龄别死亡率
Figure 5.10.5 Age-specific mortality rates of lung cancer in urban areas of Beijing, 2019

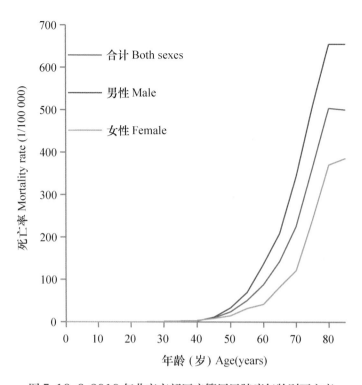

图 5.10.6 2019 年北京市郊区户籍居民肺癌年龄别死亡率
Figure 5.10.6 Age-specific mortality rates of lung cancer in peri-urban areas of Beijing, 2019

2019 年，北京市肺癌世标发病率和死亡率在 16 个辖区间有一定差异，郊区发病率和死亡率均高于城区（图 5.10.7，图 5.10.8）。

In 2019, there were some differences among the 16 districts in ASR World for incidence and mortality of lung cancer in Beijing. The incidence and mortality rates were higher in peri-urban areas than in urban areas（Figure 5.10.7-5.10.8）.

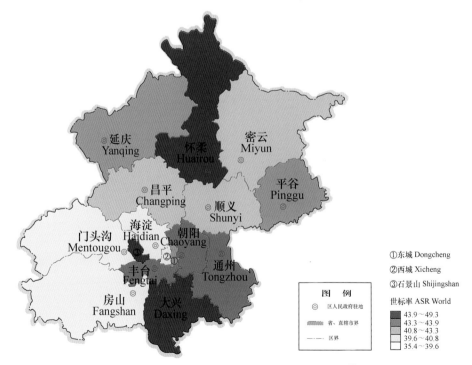

图 5.10.7 2019 年北京市户籍居民肺癌世标发病率（1/10⁵）地区分布情况
Figure 5.10.7 ASRs World for incidence of lung cancer（1/10⁵）by district in Beijing, 2019

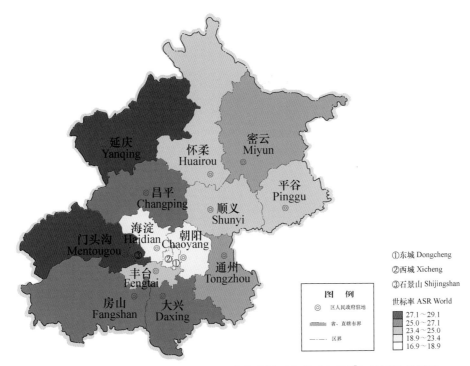

图 5.10.8 2019 年北京市户籍居民肺癌世标死亡率（1/10^5）地区分布情况

Figure 5.10.8 ASRs World for mortality of lung cancer（1/10^5）by district in Beijing, 2019

全部肺癌新发病例中，有明确亚部位的病例占 63.19%。其中肺上叶是最常见的肺癌发病亚部位，占 56.11%；其后依次为下叶和中叶，分别占 35.19% 和 5.88%（图 5.10.9）。

About 63.19% of new cases were assigned to specified categories of lung cancer site. Among those, the upper lobe was the most common subsite, accounting for 56.11% of all cases, followed by the lower lobe（35.19%）and the middle lobe（5.88%）（Figure 5.10.9）.

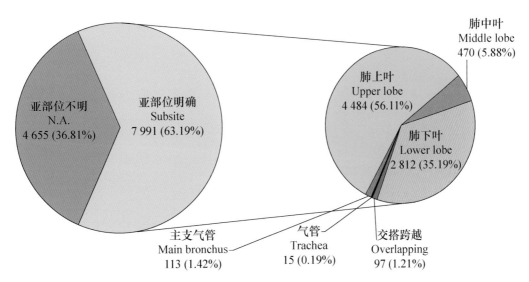

图 5.10.9 2019 年北京市户籍居民肺癌亚部位分布情况

Figure 5.10.9 Subsite distribution of lung cancer in Beijing, 2019

（撰稿 杨雷，校稿 李晴雨）

5.11 骨（C40-41）

2019 年，北京市骨癌新发病例数为 153 例，占全部恶性肿瘤发病的 0.26%，位居恶性肿瘤发病第 22 位；其中男性 88 例，女性 65 例，城区 84 例，郊区 69 例。骨癌发病率为 1.10/10 万，中标发病率为 0.72/10 万，世标发病率为 0.71/10 万；男性世标发病率为女性的 1.36 倍，郊区世标发病率为城区的 1.41 倍。0~74 岁累积发病率为 0.06%（表 5.11.1）。

5.11 Bone（C40-41）

There were 153 new cases diagnosed as bone cancer（88 males and 65 females, 84 in urban areas and 69 in peri-urban areas）, accounting for 0.26% of new cases of all cancers in 2019. Bone cancer was the 22nd common cancer in Beijing. The crude incidence rate was 1.10 per 100,000, with an ASR China and an ASR World of 0.72 and 0.71 per 100,000, respectively. The ASR World for incidence was 36% higher in males than in females and 41% higher in peri-urban areas than in urban areas. The cumulative incidence rate for subjects aged 0 to 74 years was 0.06%（Table 5.11.1）.

表 5.11.1 2019 年北京市户籍居民骨癌发病情况
Table 5.11.1 Incidence of bone cancer in Beijing, 2019

地区 Area	性别 Sex	例数 No. of cases	粗率 Crude rate （1/10⁵）	构成比 Freq.（%）	中标率 ASR China （1/10⁵）	世标率 ASR World （1/10⁵）	累积率 Cumulative rate（0~74, %）	顺位 Rank
全市 All areas	合计 Both	153	1.10	0.26	0.72	0.71	0.06	22
	男性 Male	88	1.28	0.31	0.84	0.82	0.07	18
	女性 Female	65	0.93	0.22	0.62	0.60	0.06	20
城区 Urban areas	合计 Both	84	0.98	0.22	0.61	0.62	0.06	22
	男性 Male	44	1.04	0.24	0.55	0.61	0.05	19
	女性 Female	40	0.93	0.20	0.68	0.64	0.06	20
郊区 Peri-urban areas	合计 Both	69	1.30	0.34	0.93	0.88	0.07	21
	男性 Male	44	1.66	0.44	1.30	1.18	0.10	17
	女性 Female	25	0.94	0.25	0.56	0.57	0.05	19

2019 年，北京市骨癌死亡病例数为 94 例，占全部恶性肿瘤死亡的 0.34%，位居恶性肿瘤死亡第 22 位；其中男性 60 例，女性 34 例，城区 56 例，郊区 38 例。骨癌死亡率为 0.68/10 万，中标死亡率为 0.38/10 万，世标死亡率为 0.36/10 万；男性世标死亡率为女性的 1.64 倍，郊区世标死亡率为城区的 1.27 倍。0~74 岁累积死亡率为 0.03%（表 5.11.2）。

A total of 94 cases died of bone cancer（60 males and 34 females, 56 in urban areas and 38 in peri-urban areas）, accounting for 0.34% of all cancer deaths in 2019. Bone cancer was the 22nd leading cause of cancer deaths in all cancers. The crude mortality rate was 0.68 per 100,000, with an ASR China and an ASR World of 0.38 and 0.36 per 100,000, respectively. The ASR World for mortality was 64% higher in males than in females and 27% higher in peri-urban areas than in urban areas. The cumulative mortality rate for subjects aged 0 to 74 years was 0.03%（Table 5.11.2）.

表 5.11.2 2019 年北京市户籍居民骨癌死亡情况
Table 5.11.2 Mortality of bone cancer in Beijing, 2019

地区 Area	性别 Sex	例数 No. of deaths	粗率 Crude rate （1/10⁵）	构成比 Freq.（%）	中标率 ASR China （1/10⁵）	世标率 ASR World （1/10⁵）	累积率 Cumulative rate（0~74, %）	顺位 Rank
全市 All areas	合计 Both	94	0.68	0.34	0.38	0.36	0.03	22
	男性 Male	60	0.87	0.37	0.49	0.45	0.04	18
	女性 Female	34	0.49	0.31	0.29	0.28	0.02	21
城区 Urban areas	合计 Both	56	0.66	0.31	0.36	0.33	0.03	23
	男性 Male	34	0.80	0.33	0.45	0.42	0.03	18
	女性 Female	22	0.51	0.29	0.27	0.25	0.02	21
郊区 Peri-urban areas	合计 Both	38	0.71	0.40	0.44	0.42	0.04	20
	男性 Male	26	0.98	0.45	0.55	0.51	0.05	16
	女性 Female	12	0.45	0.33	0.34	0.34	0.03	19

北京市骨癌世标发病率 2010 年为 0.73/10 万，2019 年为 0.71/10 万，年均变化百分比为 -0.91%（$P = 0.642$）；男性和女性世标发病率 10 年间年均变化百分比分别为 0.28%（$P =$

The ASR World for incidence of bone cancer was 0.73 per 100,000 in 2010 and 0.71 per 100,000 in 2019; and the APC of ASR World for incidence was -0.91%（$P = 0.642$）. The APCs of ASR World for incidence of bone cancer in males and females

0.903）和 -2.52%（*P*=0.248）。北京市骨癌
世标死亡率2010年为0.43/10万，2019年为
0.36/10万，年均变化百分比为 -0.87%（*P*=
0.486）；男性和女性世标死亡率10年间年均
变化百分比分别为 -1.19%（*P*=0.344）和
-0.18%（*P*=0.949）。

骨癌年龄别发病率和死亡率波动较大，在55
岁之前处于均较低水平，55岁之后开始迅速上升
（图5.11.1至图5.11.6）。男性的发病率和死亡率
均在85岁及以上年龄组达到高峰，女性的发病率
和死亡率均在80～84岁组达到高峰（图5.11.1和
图5.11.4）。城区和郊区年龄别发病率、死亡率变
化有一定差异，但总体趋势相同（图5.11.2和图
5.11.3，图5.11.5和图5.11.6）。

were 0.28%（*P*=0.903）and -2.52%（*P*=0.248），respectively. The ASR World for mortality of bone cancer was 0.43 per 100,000 in 2010 and 0.36 per 100,000 in 2019; and the APC of ASR World for mortality was -0.87%（*P*=0.486）. The APCs of ASR World for mortality of bone cancer in males and females were -1.19%（*P*=0.344）and -0.18%（*P*=0.949），respectively.

The age-specific incidence and mortality rates of bone cancer showed wide fluctuations. The rates were relatively low in people below 55 years old and increased dramatically in people older than that（Figure 5.11.1-5.11.6）. The age-specific incidence and mortality rates for males peaked at the age group of 85 years and above, while the age-specific incidence and mortality rates for females peaked at the age group of 80-84 years（Figure 5.11.1, Figure 5.11.4）. There were some differences in age-specific incidence and mortality rates between urban and peri-urban areas, but the overall trends were same（Figure 5.11.2-5.11.3, Figure 5.11.5-5.11.6）.

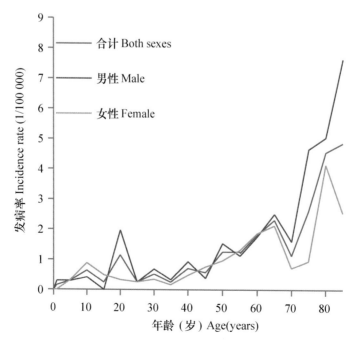

图 5.11.1 2019 年北京市户籍居民骨癌年龄别发病率
Figure 5.11.1 Age-specific incidence rates of bone cancer in Beijing, 2019

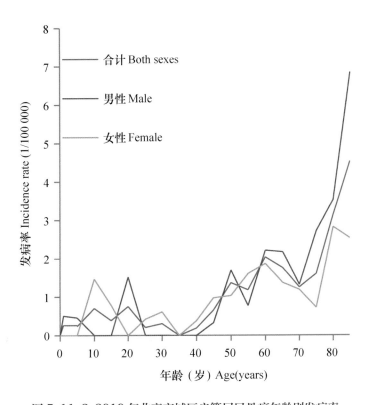

图 5.11.2 2019 年北京市城区户籍居民骨癌年龄别发病率
Figure 5.11.2 Age-specific incidence rates of bone cancer in urban areas of Beijing, 2019

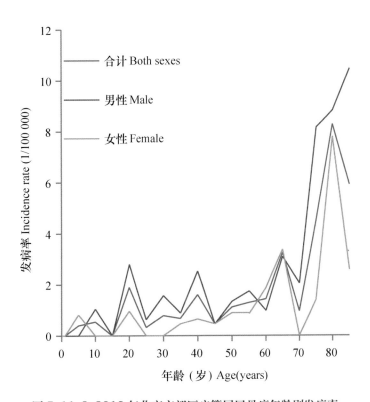

图 5.11.3 2019 年北京市郊区户籍居民骨癌年龄别发病率
Figure 5.11.3 Age-specific incidence rates of bone cancer in peri-urban areas of Beijing, 2019

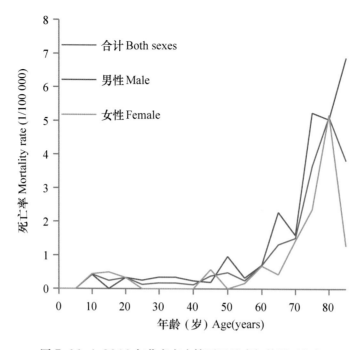

图 5.11.4 2019 年北京市户籍居民骨癌年龄别死亡率
Figure 5.11.4 Age-specific mortality rates of bone cancer in Beijing, 2019

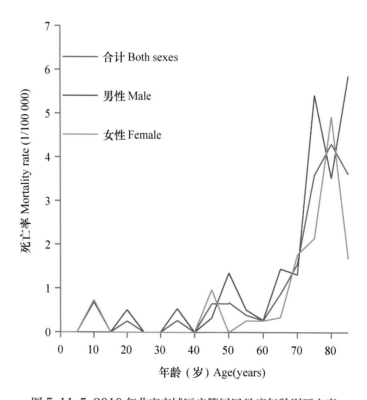

图 5.11.5 2019 年北京市城区户籍居民骨癌年龄别死亡率
Figure 5.11.5 Age-specific mortality rates of bone cancer in urban areas of Beijing, 2019

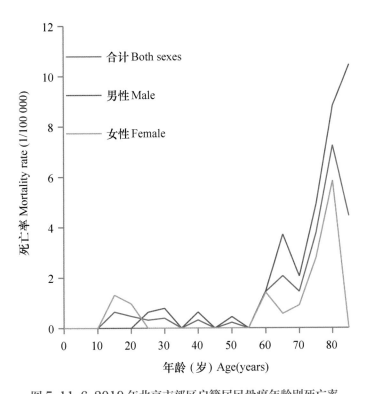

图 5.11.6 2019 年北京市郊区户籍居民骨癌年龄别死亡率

Figure 5.11.6 Age-specific mortality rates of bone cancer in peri-urban areas of Beijing, 2019

全部骨癌新发病例中，28.10% 的骨癌发生在四肢的骨和关节软骨，71.90% 发生在其他和未特指部位的骨和关节软骨（图 5.11.7）。

For subsites, about 28.10% of bone cancer occurred in the bone and articular cartilage of limbs, and 71.90% developed in the bone and articular cartilage of other and unspecified sites (Figure 5.11.7) .

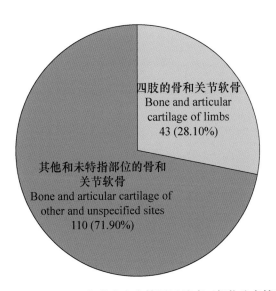

图 5.11.7 2019 年北京市户籍居民骨癌亚部位分布情况

Figure 5.11.7 Subsite distribution of bone cancer in Beijing, 2019

（撰稿 李晴雨，校稿 刘硕）

5.12 女性乳腺（C50）

　　2019 年，北京市女性乳腺癌新发病例数为 5 949 例，占女性全部恶性肿瘤发病的 20.06%，位居女性恶性肿瘤发病第 1 位；其中城区 4 098 例，郊区 1 851 例。女性乳腺癌发病率为 85.33/10 万，中标发病率为 52.17/10 万，世标发病率为 48.92/10 万；城区世标发病率为郊区的 1.27 倍。0~74 岁累积发病率为 5.37%（表 5.12.1）。

5.12 Female breast（C50）

There were 5,949 new cases diagnosed as female breast cancer（4,098 in urban areas and 1,851 in peri-urban areas）, accounting for 20.06% of new cases of all cancers among females in 2019. Breast cancer was the most common cancer among females in Beijing. The crude incidence rate was 85.33 per 100,000, with an ASR China and an ASR World of 52.17 and 48.92 per 100,000, respectively. The ASR World for incidence was 27% higher in urban areas than in peri-urban areas. The cumulative incidence rate for subjects aged 0 to 74 years was 5.37%（Table 5.12.1）.

表 5.12.1　2019 年北京市户籍居民女性乳腺癌发病情况
Table 5.12.1 Incidence of female breast cancer in Beijing, 2019

地区 Area	例数 No. of cases	粗率 Crude rate （1/10^5）	构成比 Freq.（%）	中标率 ASR China （1/10^5）	世标率 ASR World （1/10^5）	累积率 Cumulative rate（0~74, %）	顺位 Rank
全市 All areas	5 949	85.33	20.06	52.17	48.92	5.37	1
城区 Urban areas	4 098	95.27	20.94	56.32	53.18	5.91	1
郊区 Peri-urban areas	1 851	69.32	18.34	45.33	41.89	4.51	2

　　2019 年，北京市女性乳腺癌死亡病例数为 1 167 例，占女性全部恶性肿瘤死亡的 10.47%，位居女性恶性肿瘤死亡第 3 位；其中城区 864 例，郊区 303 例。女性乳腺癌死亡率为 16.74/10 万，中标死亡率为 7.38/10 万，世标死亡率为 7.23/10 万；城区世标死亡率为郊区的 1.38 倍。0~74 岁累积死亡率为 0.77%（表 5.12.2）。

A total of 1,167 female cases died of breast cancer（864 in urban areas and 303 in peri-urban areas）, accounting for 10.47% of all cancer deaths among females in 2019. Female breast cancer was the 3rd leading cause of cancer deaths in all cancers among females. The crude mortality rate was 16.74 per 100,000, with an ASR China and an ASR World of 7.38 and 7.23 per 100,000, respectively. The ASR World for mortality in urban areas was 38% higher than that in peri-urban areas. The cumulative mortality rate for subjects aged 0 to 74 years was 0.77%（Table 5.12.2）.

表 5.12.2 2019 年北京市户籍居民女性乳腺癌死亡情况
Table 5.12.2 Mortality of female breast cancer in Beijing, 2019

地区 Area	例数 No. of deaths	粗率 Crude rate (1/10^5)	构成比 Freq.（%）	中标率 ASR China (1/10^5)	世标率 ASR World (1/10^5)	累积率 Cumulative rate (0~74, %)	顺位 Rank
全市 All areas	1 167	16.74	10.47	7.38	7.23	0.77	3
城区 Urban areas	864	20.09	11.55	8.08	7.97	0.84	3
郊区 Peri-urban areas	303	11.35	8.27	6.02	5.79	0.66	3

北京市女性乳腺癌世标发病率由 2010 年的 35.59/10 万上升到 2019 年的 48.92/10 万，年均变化百分比为 2.89%（$P < 0.001$）；女性乳腺癌世标死亡率 2010 年为 6.96/10 万，2019 年为 7.23/10 万，年均变化百分比为 0.35%（$P = 0.132$）。

女性乳腺癌发病率自 25～29 岁组开始快速升高，至 45～49 岁组达到第一个高峰后有所下降，在 60～64 岁组达到第二个高峰，整体呈现明显的"双峰分布"。女性乳腺癌年龄别死亡率自 40～44 岁组开始快速升高，在 85 岁及以上年龄组达到高峰。城区和郊区年龄别发病率、死亡率有一定差异（图 5.12.1 至图 5.12.6）。

The ASR World for incidence of female breast cancer increased from 35.59 per 100,000 in 2010 to 48.92 per 100,000 in 2019; and the APC of ASR World for incidence was 2.89% ($P < 0.001$). The ASR World for mortality of female breast cancer were 6.96 and 7.23 per 100,000 in 2010 and 2019 respectively; and the APC of ASR World for mortality was 0.35% ($P = 0.132$).

The age-specific incidence rate of female breast cancer showed a double-peak pattern. The rate increased dramatically from the age group of 25-29 years, and the first peak appeared at the age group of 45-49 years, after which the rates decreased and peaked at the age group of 60-64 years again. The age-specific mortality rate of female breast cancer increased sharply at the age group of 40-44 years, and peaked at the age group of 85 years and above. There were some differences in age-specific incidence and mortality rates between urban and peri-urban areas (Figure 5.12.1-5.12.6).

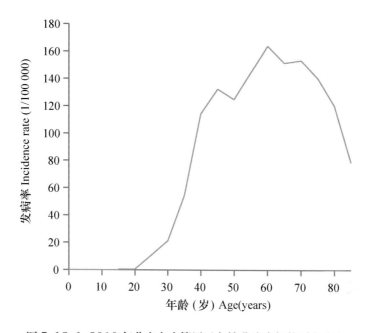

图 5.12.1 2019 年北京市户籍居民女性乳腺癌年龄别发病率
Figure 5.12.1 Age-specific incidence rates of female breast cancer in Beijing, 2019

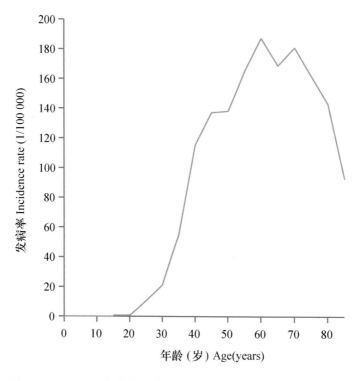

图 5.12.2 2019 年北京市城区户籍居民女性乳腺癌年龄别发病率
Figure5.12.2 Age-specific incidence rates of female breast cancer in urban areas of Beijing, 2019

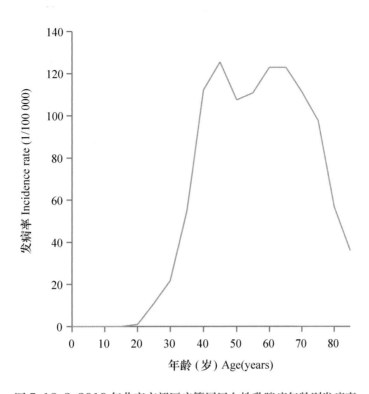

图 5.12.3　2019 年北京市郊区户籍居民女性乳腺癌年龄别发病率

Figure 5.12.3 Age-specific incidence rates of female breast cancer in peri-urban areas of Beijing, 2019

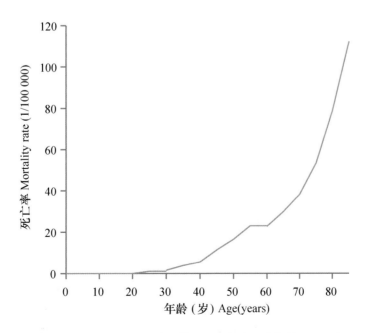

图 5.12.4　2019 年北京市户籍居民女性乳腺癌年龄别死亡率

Figure 5.12.4 Age-specific mortality rates of female breast cancer in Beijing, 2019

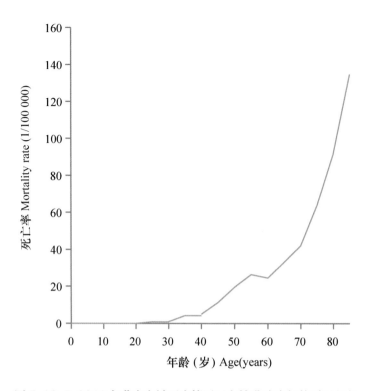

图 5.12.5 2019 年北京市城区户籍居民女性乳腺癌年龄别死亡率
Figure 5.12.5 Age-specific mortality rates of female breast cancer in urban areas of Beijing, 2019

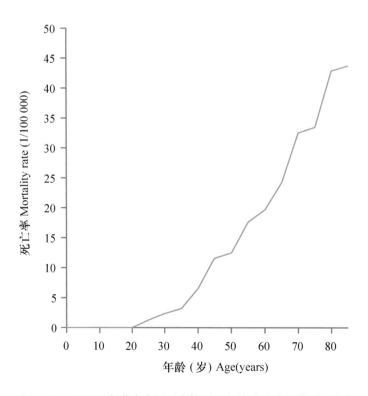

图 5.12.6 2019 年北京市郊区户籍居民女性乳腺癌年龄别死亡率
Figure 5.12.6 Age-specific mortality rates of female breast cancer in peri-urban areas of Beijing, 2019

2019 年，北京市女性乳腺癌世标发病率和死亡率在 16 个辖区间有显著差异，城区发病率和死亡率均高于郊区（图 5.12.7 和图 5.12.8）。

In 2019, there were significant differences among the 16 districts in ASR World for incidence and mortality of female breast cancer in Beijing. The incidence and mortality rates were higher in urban areas than in peri-urban areas（Figure 5.12.7-5.12.8）.

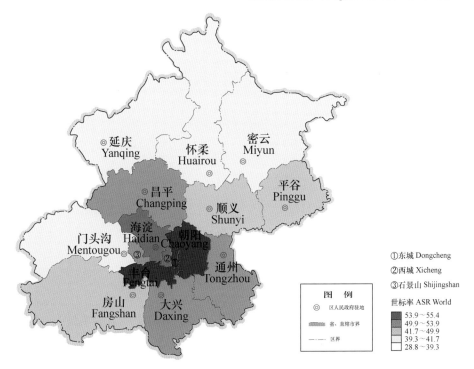

图 5.12.7 2019 年北京市户籍居民女性乳腺癌世标发病率（1/10⁵）地区分布情况
Figure 5.12.7 ASRs World for incidence of female breast cancer（1/10⁵）by district in Beijing, 2019

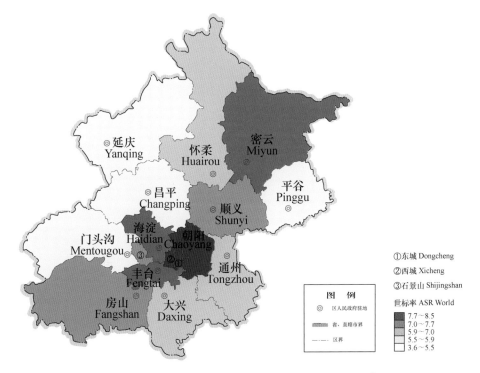

图 5.12.8 2019 年北京市户籍居民女性乳腺癌世标死亡率（1/10⁵）地区分布情况
Figure 5.12.8 ASRs World for mortality of female breast cancer（1/10⁵）by district in Beijing, 2019

全部女性乳腺癌新发病例中,有明确亚部位的病例占70.73%。其中乳腺上外象限是最常见的发病部位,占45.89%;其后依次为上内象限(19.01%)、交搭跨越(14.40%)、下外象限(10.86%)、下内象限(6.58%)、中央部(2.12%)、乳头和乳晕(1.12%)以及腋尾部(0.02%)(图5.12.9)。

About 70.73% of new cases were assigned to specified categories of female breast cancer site. Among those, the upper outer quadrant of breast was the most common site, accounting for 45.89% of all cases, followed by the upper inner (19.01%), the overlapping (14.40%), the lower outer (10.86%), the lower inner (6.58%), the central portion (2.12%), the nipple and areola (1.12%), and the axillary tail (0.02%) (Figure 5.12.9).

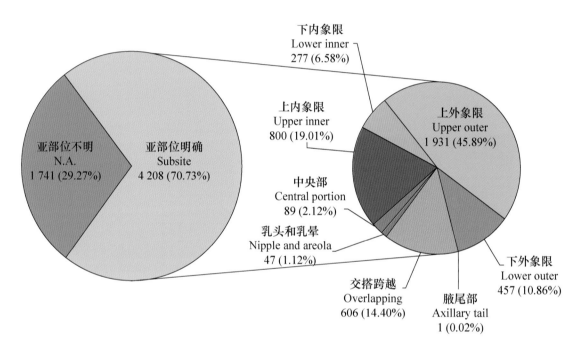

图 5.12.9 2019 年北京市户籍居民女性乳腺癌亚部位分布情况
Figure 5.12.9 Subsite distribution of female breast cancer in Beijing, 2019

(撰稿 刘硕,校稿 李浩鑫)

5.13 子宫颈（C53）

2019 年，北京市子宫颈癌新发病例数为 659 例，占女性全部恶性肿瘤发病的 2.22%，位居女性恶性肿瘤发病第 11 位；其中城区 402 例，郊区 257 例。子宫颈癌发病率为 9.45/10 万，中标发病率为 6.65/10 万，世标发病率为 5.94/10 万；郊区世标发病率为城区的 1.02 倍。0~74 岁累积发病率为 0.61%（表 5.13.1）。

5.13 Cervix（C53）

There were 659 new cases diagnosed as cervical cancer（402 in urban areas and 257 in peri-urban areas）, accounting for 2.22% of new female cases of all cancers in 2019. Cervical cancer was the 11th common female cancer in Beijing. The crude incidence rate was 9.45 per 100,000, with an ASR China and an ASR World of 6.65 and 5.94 per 100,000, respectively. The ASR World for incidence was 2% higher in peri-urban areas than in urban areas. The cumulative incidence rate for subjects aged 0 to 74 years was 0.61%（Table 5.13.1）.

表 5.13.1　2019 年北京市户籍居民子宫颈癌发病情况
Table 5.13.1 Incidence of cervical cancer in Beijing, 2019

地区 Area	例数 No. of cases	粗率 Crude rate （1/10^5）	构成比 Freq.（%）	中标率 ASR China （1/10^5）	世标率 ASR World （1/10^5）	累积率 Cumulative rate（0~74, %）	顺位 Rank
全市 All areas	659	9.45	2.22	6.65	5.94	0.61	11
城区 Urban areas	402	9.35	2.05	6.54	5.92	0.61	11
郊区 Peri-urban areas	257	9.62	2.55	6.89	6.01	0.60	9

2019 年，北京市子宫颈癌死亡病例数为 244 例，占女性全部恶性肿瘤死亡的 2.19%，位居女性恶性肿瘤死亡第 13 位；其中城区 143 例，郊区 101 例。子宫颈癌死亡率为 3.50/10 万，中标死亡率为 1.91/10 万，世标死亡率为 1.81/10 万；郊区世标死亡率为城区的 1.13 倍。0~74 岁累积死亡率为 0.18%（表 5.13.2）。

A total of 244 cases died of cervical cancer（143 in urban areas and 101 in peri-urban areas）, accounting for 2.19% of all female cancer deaths in 2019. Cervical cancer was the 13th leading cause of cancer deaths in all cancers among females. The crude mortality rate was 3.50 per 100,000, with an ASR China and an ASR World of 1.91 and 1.81 per 100,000, respectively. The ASR World for mortality was 13% higher in peri-urban areas than in urban areas. The cumulative mortality rate for subjects aged 0 to 74 years was 0.18%（Table 5.13.2）.

表 5.13.2 2019 年北京市户籍居民子宫颈癌死亡情况
Table 5.13.2 Mortality of cervical cancer in Beijing, 2019

地区 Area	例数 No. of deaths	粗率 Crude rate （1/10⁵）	构成比 Freq.（%）	中标率 ASR China （1/10⁵）	世标率 ASR World （1/10⁵）	累积率 Cumulative rate（0~74, %）	顺位 Rank
全市 All areas	244	3.50	2.19	1.91	1.81	0.18	13
城区 Urban areas	143	3.32	1.91	1.86	1.75	0.17	14
郊区 Peri-urban areas	101	3.78	2.76	2.05	1.97	0.19	12

北京市子宫颈癌世标发病率2010年为5.34/10万，2019年为5.94/10万，年均变化百分比为0.75%（P=0.311）。北京市子宫颈癌世标死亡率由2010年的1.57/10万上升到2019年的1.81/10万，年均变化百分比为2.33%（P=0.029）。

子宫颈癌年龄别发病率在25岁以前处于较低水平，随后快速上升，至45~49岁年龄组达高峰，之后逐渐下降（图5.13.1）。年龄别死亡率在35岁以前处于较低水平，35岁以后随年龄的增长逐渐升高，在60~64岁年龄组出现一个小高峰，随后降低，70岁之后再次迅速上升，至85岁及以上年龄组达到高峰（图5.13.4）。城区和郊区年龄别发病率、死亡率变化有一定差异，但总体趋势相同，郊区波动较为明显（图5.13.2和图5.13.3，图5.13.5和图5.13.6）。

The ASR World for incidence of cervical cancer increased from 5.34 per 100,000 in 2010 to 5.94 per 100,000 in 2019; and the APC of ASR World for incidence was 0.75%（P=0.311）. The ASR World for mortality of cervical cancer increased from 1.57 per 100,000 in 2010 to 1.81 per 100,000 in 2019; and the APC of ASR World for mortality was 2.33%（P=0.029）.

The age-specific incidence rates of cervical cancer were relatively low in people below 25 years old, and increased sharply in people older than that（Figure 5.13.1）. It peaked at the age group of 45-49 years, and then decreased gradually. The age-specific mortality rates of cervical cancer were low in people below 35 years old and gradually increased with age. The first peak appeared at the age group of 60-64 years, after which the rate decreased before 70 years old. But it increased dramatically since then, reaching the second peak at the age group of 85 years and above（Figure 5.13.4）. There were some differences in age-specific incidence and mortality rates between urban and peri-urban areas, but the overall trends were same. The age-specific incidence and mortality rates in peri-urban areas showed huge fluctuations（Figure 5.13.2-5.13.3, Figure 5.13.5-5.13.6）.

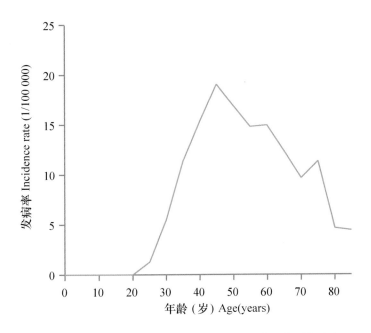

图 5.13.1 2019 年北京市户籍居民子宫颈癌年龄别发病率
Figure 5.13.1 Age-specific incidence rates of cervical cancer in Beijing, 2019

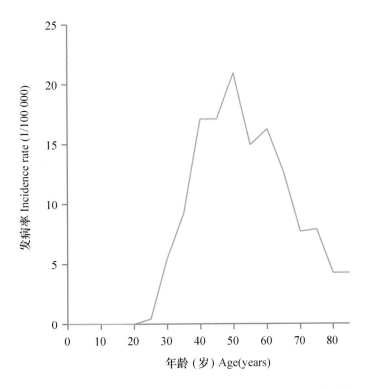

图 5.13.2 2019 年北京市城区户籍居民子宫颈癌年龄别发病率
Figure 5.13.2 Age-specific incidence rates of cervical cancer in urban areas of Beijing, 2019

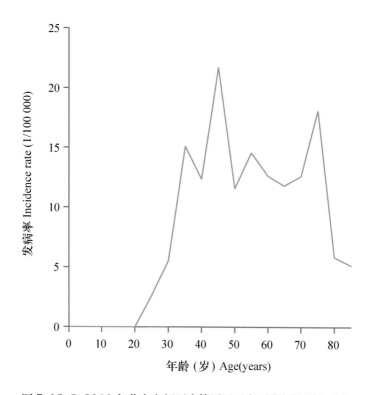

图 5.13.3　2019 年北京市郊区户籍居民子宫颈癌年龄别发病率
Figure 5.13.3　Age-specific incidence rates of cervical cancer in peri-urban areas of Beijing, 2019

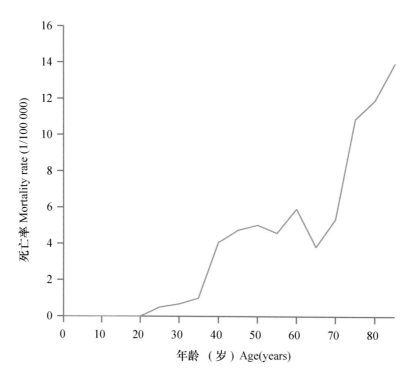

图 5.13.4　2019 年北京市户籍居民子宫颈癌年龄别死亡率
Figure 5.13.4　Age-specific mortality rates of cervical cancer in Beijing, 2019

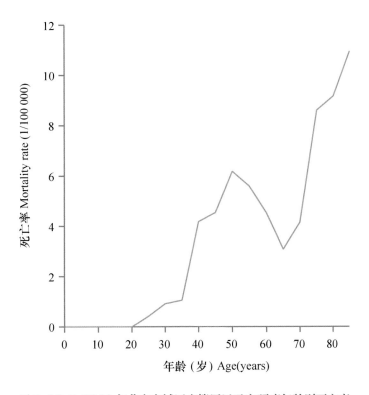

图 5.13.5 2019 年北京市城区户籍居民子宫颈癌年龄别死亡率
Figure 5.13.5 Age-specific mortality rates of cervical cancer in urban areas of Beijing, 2019

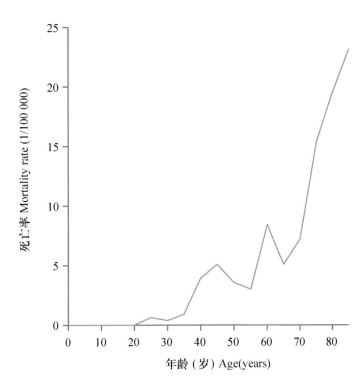

图 5.13.6 2019 年北京市郊区户籍居民子宫颈癌年龄别死亡率
Figure 5.13.6 Age-specific mortality rates of cervical cancer in peri-urban areas of Beijing, 2019

2019年，北京市子宫颈癌世标发病率和死亡率在16个辖区间存在一定差异，郊区发病率和死亡率均高于城区（图5.13.7和图5.13.8）。

In 2019, there were some differences among the 16 districts in ASR World for incidence and mortality of cervical cancer in Beijing. The incidence and mortality rates were higher in peri-urban areas than in urban areas（Figure 5.13.7-5.13.8）.

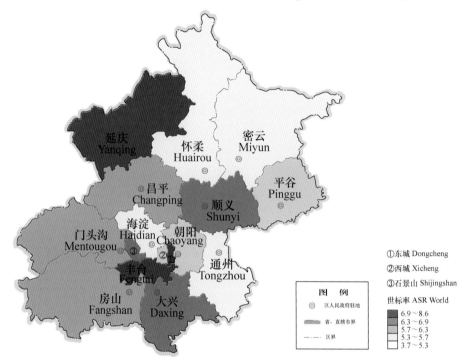

图 5.13.7 2019 年北京市户籍居民子宫颈癌世标发病率（1/10⁵）地区分布情况

Figure 5.13.7 ASRs World for incidence of cervical cancer（1/10⁵）by district in Beijing, 2019

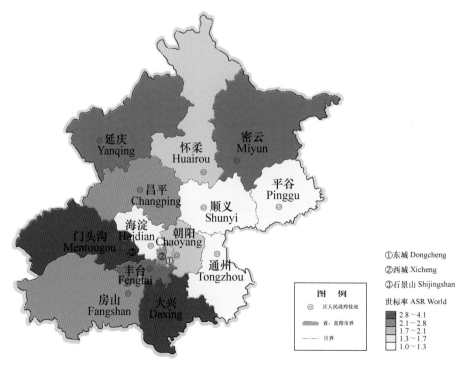

图 5.13.8 2019 年北京市户籍居民子宫颈癌世标死亡率（1/10⁵）地区分布情况

Figure 5.13.8 ASRs World for mortality of cervical cancer（1/10⁵）by district in Beijing, 2019

（撰稿 张希，校稿 李浩鑫）

5.14 子宫体（C54-55）

2019 年，北京市子宫体癌新发病例数为 1 523 例，占女性全部恶性肿瘤发病的 5.13%，位居女性恶性肿瘤发病第 5 位；其中城区 977 例，郊区 546 例。子宫体癌发病率为 21.85/10 万，中标发病率为 12.79/10 万，世标发病率为 12.38/10 万；城区世标发病率为郊区的 1.07 倍。0~74 岁累积发病率为 1.43%（表 5.14.1）。

5.14 Uterus（C54-55）

There were 1,523 new cases diagnosed as uterus cancer（977 in urban areas and 546 in peri-urban areas）, accounting for 5.13% of new cases of all cancers among females in 2019. Uterus cancer was the 5th common female cancer in Beijing. The crude incidence rate was 21.85 per 100,000, with an ASR China and an ASR World of 12.79 and 12.38 per 100,000, respectively. The ASR World for incidence was 7% higher in urban areas than in peri-urban areas. The cumulative incidence rate for subjects aged 0 to 74 years was 1.43%（Table 5.14.1）.

表 5.14.1 2019 年北京市户籍居民子宫体癌发病情况
Table 5.14.1 Incidence of uterus cancer in Beijing, 2019

地区 Area	例数 No. of cases	粗率 Crude rate （1/10⁵）	构成比 Freq.（%）	中标率 ASR China （1/10⁵）	世标率 ASR World （1/10⁵）	累积率 Cumulative rate（0~74, %）	顺位 Rank
全市 All areas	1 523	21.85	5.13	12.79	12.38	1.43	5
城区 Urban areas	977	22.71	4.99	13.14	12.73	1.49	5
郊区 Peri-urban areas	546	20.45	5.41	12.29	11.88	1.34	5

2019 年，北京市子宫体癌死亡病例数为 239 例，占女性全部恶性肿瘤死亡的 2.14%，位居女性恶性肿瘤死亡第 14 位；其中城区 163 例，郊区 76 例。子宫体癌死亡率为 3.43/10 万，中标死亡率为 1.53/10 万，世标死亡率为 1.51/10 万；城区世标死亡率为郊区的 1.16 倍。0~74 岁累积死亡率为 0.19%（表 5.14.2）。

A total of 239 cases died of uterus cancer（163 in urban areas and 76 in peri-urban areas）, accounting for 2.14% of all female cancer deaths in 2019. Uterus cancer was the 14th leading cause of cancer deaths in all cancers among females. The crude mortality rate was 3.43 per 100,000, with an ASR China and an ASR World of 1.53 and 1.51 per 100,000, respectively. The ASR World for mortality in urban areas were 16% higher than that in peri-urban areas. The cumulative mortality rate for subjects aged 0 to 74 years was 0.19%（Table 5.14.2）.

表 5.14.2 2019 年北京市户籍居民子宫体癌死亡情况
Table 5.14.2 Mortality of uterus cancer in Beijing, 2019

地区 Area	例数 No. of deaths	粗率 Crude rate （1/10⁵）	构成比 Freq.（%）	中标率 ASR China （1/10⁵）	世标率 ASR World （1/10⁵）	累积率 Cumulative rate（0~74, %）	顺位 Rank
全市 All areas	239	3.43	2.14	1.53	1.51	0.19	14
城区 Urban areas	163	3.79	2.18	1.60	1.58	0.20	12
郊区 Peri-urban areas	76	2.85	2.07	1.40	1.36	0.17	15

北京市子宫体癌世标发病率由 2010 年的 8.25/10 万上升到 2019 年的 12.38/10 万，10 年间年均变化百分比为 3.97%（$P < 0.001$）。北京市子宫体癌世标死亡率 2010 年为 1.68/10 万，2019 年为 1.51/10 万，年均变化百分比为 0.27%（$P = 0.781$）。

子宫体癌年龄别发病率自 20 岁开始逐渐上升，30 岁以后快速上升，至 55~59 岁年龄组达高峰，之后逐渐下降（图 5.14.1）。年龄别死亡率在 40 岁以前处于较低水平，40 岁以后随年龄的增长逐渐升高，在 80~84 岁年龄组达到高峰（图 5.14.4）。城区和郊区年龄别发病率、死亡率变化有一定差异，但总体趋势相同，郊区波动较为明显（图 5.14.2 和图 5.14.3，图 5.14.5 和图 5.14.6）。

The ASR World for incidence of uterus cancer increased from 8.25 per 100,000 in 2010 to 12.38 per 100,000 in 2019; and the APC of ASR World for incidence was 3.97%（$P < 0.001$）. The ASR World for mortality of uterus cancer was 1.68 per 100,000 in 2010 and 1.51 per 100,000 in 2019; and the APC of ASR World for mortality was 0.27%（$P = 0.781$）.

The age-specific incidence rates of uterus cancer increased gradually in people aged 20 years old, and went up rapidly in people aged 30 years and above, peaking at the age group of 55-59 years with a gradual decline thereafter（Figure 5.14.1）. The age-specific mortality rate of uterus cancer was low before 40 years old and gradually increased with advancing of age, peaking at the age group of 80-84 years（Figure 5.14.4）. There were some differences in age-specific incidence and mortality rates between urban and peri-urban areas, but the overall trends were same. The age-specific incidence and mortality rates in peri-urban areas showed huge fluctuations（Figure 5.14.2-5.14.3, Figure 5.14.5-5.14.6）.

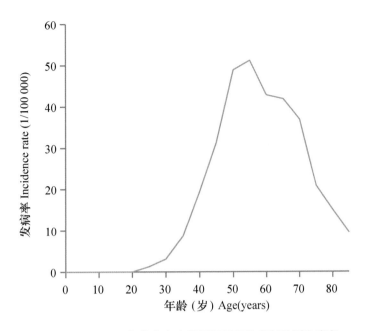

图 5.14.1 2019 年北京市户籍居民子宫体癌年龄别发病率
Figure 5.14.1 Age-specific incidence rates of uterus cancer in Beijing, 2019

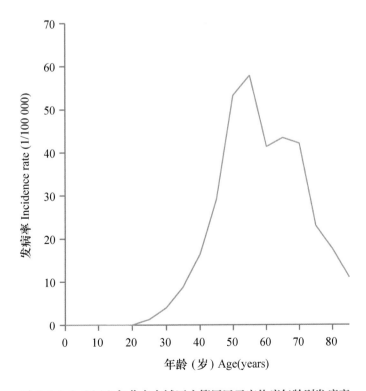

图 5.14.2 2019 年北京市城区户籍居民子宫体癌年龄别发病率
Figure 5.14.2 Age-specific incidence rates of uterus cancer in urban areas of Beijing, 2019

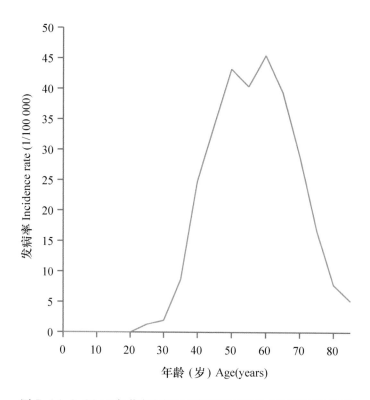

图 5.14.3 2019 年北京市郊区户籍居民子宫体癌年龄别发病率
Figure 5.14.3 Age-specific incidence rates of uterus cancer in peri-urban areas of Beijing, 2019

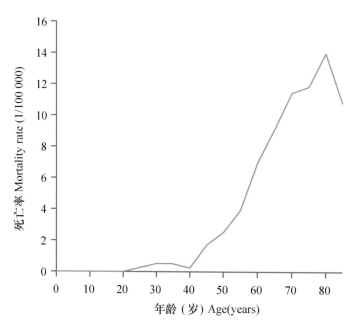

图 5.14.4 2019 年北京市户籍居民子宫体癌年龄别死亡率
Figure 5.14.4 Age-specific mortality rates of uterus cancer in Beijing, 2019

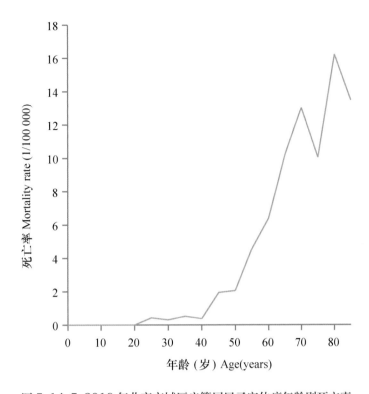

图 5.14.5 2019 年北京市城区户籍居民子宫体癌年龄别死亡率
Figure 5.14.5 Age-specific mortality rates of uterus cancer in urban areas of Beijing, 2019

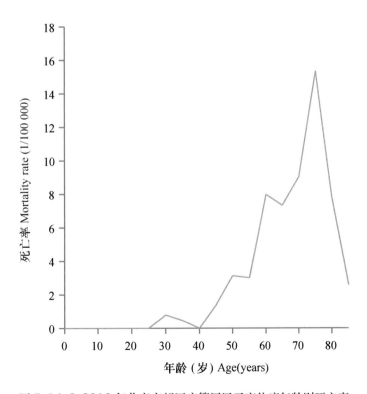

图 5.14.6 2019 年北京市郊区户籍居民子宫体癌年龄别死亡率
Figure 5.14.6 Age-specific mortality rates of uterus cancer in peri-urban areas of Beijing, 2019

2019 年，北京市子宫体癌世标发病率和死亡率在 16 个辖区间有一定差异，城区发病率和死亡率均高于郊区（图 5.14.7 和图 5.14.8）。

In 2019, there were some differences among the 16 districts in ASR World for incidence and mortality of uterus cancer in Beijing. The incidence and mortality rates of uterus cancer were higher in urban areas than in peri-urban areas（Figure 5.14.7-5.14.8）.

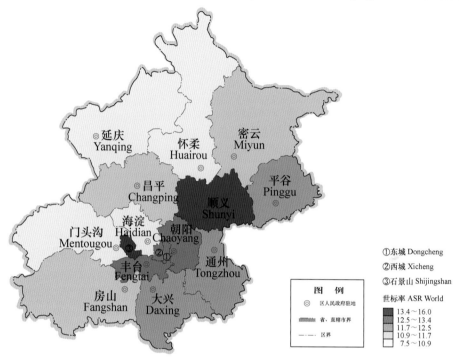

图 5.14.7 2019 年北京市户籍居民子宫体癌世标发病率（1/10^5）地区分布情况

Figure 5.14.7 ASRs World for incidence of uterus cancer（1/10^5）by district in Beijing, 2019

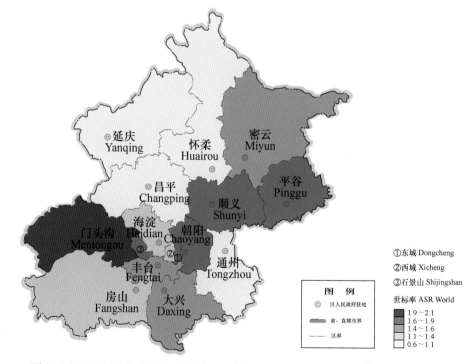

图 5.14.8 2019 年北京市户籍居民子宫体癌世标死亡率（1/10^5）地区分布情况

Figure 5.14.8 ASRs World for mortality of uterus cancer（1/10^5）by district in Beijing, 2019

（撰稿 张希，校稿 李浩鑫）

5.15 卵巢（C56）

2019 年，北京市卵巢癌新发病例数为 851 例，占女性全部恶性肿瘤发病的 2.87%，位居女性恶性肿瘤发病第 7 位；其中城区 559 例，郊区 292 例。卵巢癌发病率为 12.21/10 万，中标发病率为 7.59/10 万，世标发病率为 7.26/10 万；城区世标发病率为郊区的 1.21 倍。0~74 岁累积发病率为 0.79%（表 5.15.1）。

5.15 Ovary（C56）

There were 851 new cases diagnosed as ovarian cancer（559 in urban areas and 292 in peri-urban areas）, accounting for 2.87% of new cases of all cancers among females in 2019. Ovarian cancer was the 7th common female cancer in Beijing. The crude incidence rate was 12.21 per 100,000, with an ASR China and an ASR World of 7.59 and 7.26 per 100,000, respectively. The ASR World for incidence in urban areas were 21% higher than that in peri-urban areas. The cumulative incidence rate for subjects aged 0 to 74 years was 0.79%（Table 5.15.1）.

表 5.15.1 2019 年北京市户籍居民卵巢癌发病情况
Table5.15.1 Incidence of ovarian cancer in Beijing, 2019

地区 Area	例数 No. of cases	粗率 Crude rate （1/10⁵）	构成比 Freq.（%）	中标率 ASR China （1/10⁵）	世标率 ASR World （1/10⁵）	累积率 Cumulative rate（0~74, %）	顺位 Rank
全市 All areas	851	12.21	2.87	7.59	7.26	0.79	7
城区 Urban areas	559	13.00	2.86	8.16	7.79	0.83	8
郊区 Peri-urban areas	292	10.94	2.89	6.71	6.44	0.71	6

2019 年，北京市卵巢癌死亡病例数为 486 例，占女性全部恶性肿瘤死亡的 4.36%，位居女性恶性肿瘤死亡第 8 位；其中城区 324 例，郊区 162 例。卵巢癌死亡率为 6.97/10 万，中标死亡率为 3.28/10 万，世标死亡率为 3.27/10 万；城区世标死亡率为郊区的 1.09 倍。0~74 岁累积死亡率为 0.39%（表 5.15.2）。

A total of 486 cases died of ovarian cancer（324 in urban areas and 162 in peri-urban areas）, accounting for 4.36% of all cancer deaths among females in 2019. Ovarian cancer was the 8th leading cause of cancer deaths in all female cancers. The crude mortality rate was 6.97 per 100,000, with an ASR China and an ASR World of 3.28 and 3.27 per 100,000, respectively. The ASR World for mortality was 9% higher in urban areas than in peri-urban areas. The cumulative mortality rate for subjects aged 0 to 74 years was 0.39%（Table 5.15.2）.

表 5.15.2 2019 年北京市户籍居民卵巢癌死亡情况
Table 5.15.2 Mortality of ovarian cancer in Beijing, 2019

地区 Area	例数 No. of deaths	粗率 Crude rate (1/10⁵)	构成比 Freq.（%）	中标率 ASR China (1/10⁵)	世标率 ASR World (1/10⁵)	累积率 Cumulative rate (0~74, %)	顺位 Rank
全市 All areas	486	6.97	4.36	3.28	3.27	0.39	8
城区 Urban areas	324	7.53	4.33	3.37	3.37	0.42	7
郊区 Peri-urban areas	162	6.07	4.42	3.12	3.09	0.36	8

北京市卵巢癌世标发病率 2010 年为 7.32 /10 万，2019 年为 7.26/10 万，年均变化百分比为 0.40%（P = 0.299）。北京市卵巢癌世标死亡率 2010 年为 3.43/10 万，2019 年为 3.27/10 万，年均变化百分比为 1.14%（P = 0.210）。

卵巢癌年龄别发病率在 20 岁以前处于较低水平，自 30~34 岁组开始快速上升，至 50~54 岁组达到第一个高峰，之后呈现较高发病水平，至 75~79 岁组开始下降（图 5.15.1）。卵巢癌年龄别死亡率在 35 岁之前处于较低水平，自 35~39 岁组开始快速上升，至 85 岁及以上年龄组达高峰（图 5.15.4）。城区和郊区年龄别发病率、死亡率变化有一定差异，但总体趋势相同，郊区波动较为明显（图 5.15.2 和图 5.15.3，图 5.15.5 和图 5.15.6）。

The ASR World for incidence of ovarian cancer was 7.32 per 100,000 in 2010 and 7.26 per 100,000 in 2019; and the APC of ASR World for incidence was 0.40%（P = 0.299）. The ASR World for mortality of ovarian cancer was 3.43 per 100,000 in 2010 and 3.27 per 100,000 in 2019; and the APC of ASR World for mortality was 1.14%（P = 0.210）.

The age-specific incidence rates of ovarian cancer were relatively low in people below 20 years old, and increased sharply in people at the age group of 30-34 years. The first peak appeared at the age group of 50-54 years old, then showed a high level of incidence, and began to decline in the age group of 75-79 years old（Figure 5.15.1）. The age-specific mortality rates of ovarian cancer were relatively low in people below 35 years old, and increased sharply in people at age group of 35-39 years, peaking at the age group of 85 years and above（Figure 5.15.4）. There were some differences in age-specific incidence and mortality rates between urban and peri-urban areas, but the overall trends were same. The age-specific incidence and mortality rates in peri-urban areas showed huge fluctuations（Figure 5.15.2-5.15.3, Figure 5.15.5-5.15.6）.

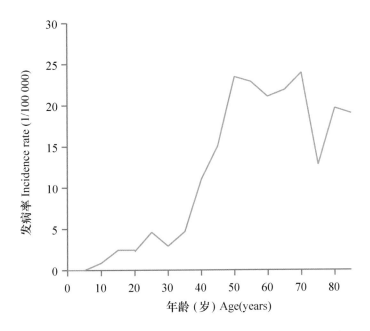

图 5.15.1 2019 年北京市户籍居民卵巢癌年龄别发病率

Figure 5.15.1 Age-specific incidence rates of ovarian cancer in Beijing, 2019

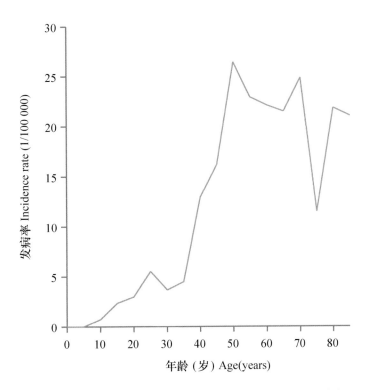

图 5.15.2 2019 年北京市城区户籍居民卵巢癌年龄别发病率

Figure 5.15.2 Age-specific incidence rates of ovarian cancer in urban areas of Beijing, 2019

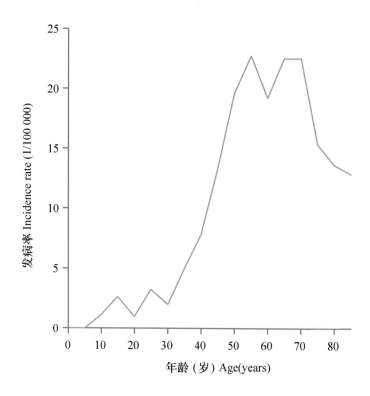

图 5.15.3 2019 年北京市郊区户籍居民卵巢癌年龄别发病率
Figure 5.15.3 Age-specific incidence rates of ovarian cancer in peri-urban areas of Beijing, 2019

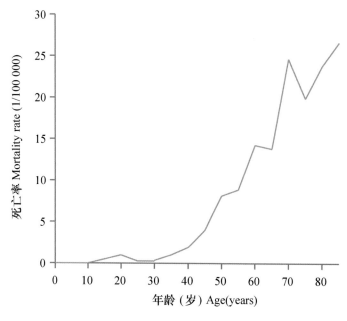

图 5.15.4 2019 年北京市户籍居民卵巢癌年龄别死亡率
Figure 5.15.4 Age-specific mortality rates of ovarian cancer in Beijing, 2019

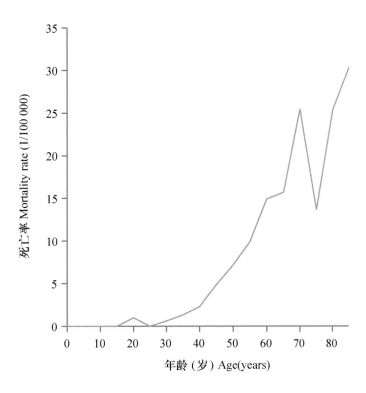

图 5.15.5 2019 年北京市城区户籍居民卵巢癌年龄别死亡率
Figure 5.15.5 Age-specific mortality rates of ovarian cancer in urban areas of Beijing, 2019

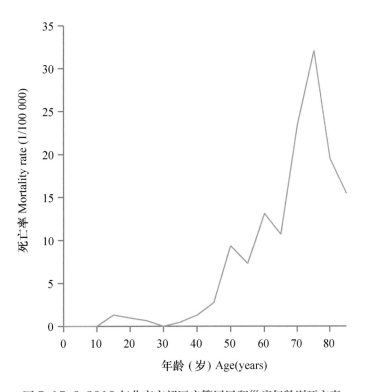

图 5.15.6 2019 年北京市郊区户籍居民卵巢癌年龄别死亡率
Figure 5.15.6 Age-specific mortality rates of ovarian cancer in peri-urban areas of Beijing, 2019

2019 年，北京市卵巢癌世标发病率和死亡率在 16 个辖区间有一定差异，城区发病率和死亡率均高于郊区（图 5.15.7 和图 5.15.8）。

In 2019, there were some differences among the 16 districts in ASR World for incidence and mortality of ovarian cancer in Beijing. The incidence and mortality rate of ovarian cancer was higher in urban areas than in peri-urban areas（Figure 5.15.7-5.15.8）.

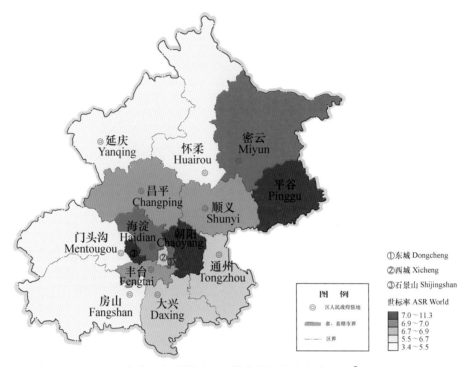

图 5.15.7 2019 年北京市户籍居民卵巢癌世标发病率（1/10^5）地区分布情况
Figure 5.15.7 ASRs World for incidence of ovarian cancer（1/10^5）by district in Beijing, 2019

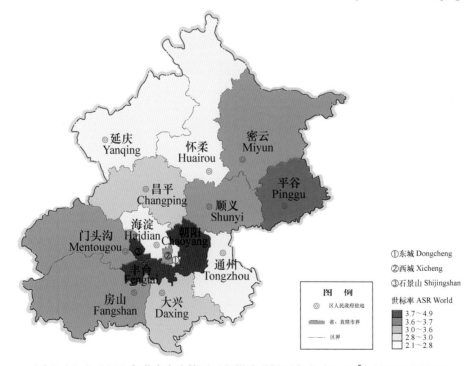

图 5.15.8 2019 年北京市户籍居民卵巢癌世标死亡率（1/10^5）地区分布情况
Figure 5.15.8 ASRs World for mortality of ovarian cancer（1/10^5）by district in Beijing, 2019

（撰稿 张希，校稿 李浩鑫）

5.16 前列腺（C61）

5.16 Prostate（C61）

2019 年，北京市前列腺癌新发病例数为 1 798 例，占男性全部恶性肿瘤发病的 6.29%，位居男性恶性肿瘤发病第 5 位；其中城区 1 337 例，郊区 461 例。前列腺癌发病率为 26.08/10 万，中标发病率为 11.04/10 万，世标发病率为 10.86/10 万；城区世标发病率为郊区的 1.55 倍。0 ~ 74 岁累积发病率为 1.33%（表 5.16.1）。

There were 1,798 new cases diagnosed as prostate cancer（1,337 in urban areas and 461 in peri-urban areas）, accounting for 6.29% of new cases of all cancers among males in 2019. Prostate cancer was the 5th common male cancer in Beijing. The crude incidence rate was 26.08 per 100,000, with an ASR China and an ASR World of 11.04 and 10.86 per 100,000, respectively. The ASR World for incidence was 55% higher in urban areas than in peri-urban areas. The cumulative incidence rate for subjects aged 0 to 74 years was 1.33%（Table 5.16.1）.

表 5.16.1 2019 年北京市户籍居民前列腺癌发病情况
Table 5.16.1 Incidence of prostate cancer in Beijing, 2019

地区 Area	例数 No. of cases	粗率 Crude rate （1/10⁵）	构成比 Freq.（%）	中标率 ASR China （1/10⁵）	世标率 ASR World （1/10⁵）	累积率 Cumulative rate（0~74, %）	顺位 Rank
全市 All areas	1 798	26.08	6.29	11.04	10.86	1.33	5
城区 Urban areas	1 337	31.52	7.23	12.65	12.45	1.55	3
郊区 Peri-urban areas	461	17.38	4.58	8.20	8.04	0.98	8

2019 年，北京市前列腺癌死亡病例数为 694 例，占男性全部恶性肿瘤死亡的 4.28%，位居男性恶性肿瘤死亡第 7 位；其中城区 517 例，郊区 177 例。前列腺癌死亡率为 10.07/10 万，中标死亡率为 3.12/10 万，世标死亡率为 3.20/10 万；城区世标死亡率为郊区的 1.14 倍。0 ~ 74 岁累积死亡率为 0.20%（表 5.16.2）。

A total of 694 cases died of prostate cancer（517 in urban areas and 177 in peri-urban areas）, accounting for 4.28% of all cancer deaths among males in 2019. Prostate cancer was the 7th leading cause of cancer deaths in all male cancers. The crude mortality rate was 10.07 per 100,000, with an ASR China and an ASR World of 3.12 and 3.20 per 100,000, respectively. The ASR World for mortality in urban areas was 14% higher than that in peri-urban areas. The cumulative mortality rate for subjects aged 0 to 74 years was 0.20%（Table 5.16.2）.

表 5.16.2　2019 年北京市户籍居民前列腺癌死亡情况
Table 5.16.2 Mortality of prostate cancer in Beijing, 2019

地区 Area	例数 No. of deaths	粗率 Crude rate （1/10^5）	构成比 Freq.（%）	中标率 ASR China （1/10^5）	世标率 ASR World （1/10^5）	累积率 Cumulative rate（0~74, %）	顺位 Rank
全市 All areas	694	10.07	4.28	3.12	3.20	0.20	7
城区 Urban areas	517	12.19	4.99	3.25	3.31	0.20	5
郊区 Peri-urban areas	177	6.67	3.03	2.81	2.89	0.21	11

北京市前列腺癌世标发病率由 2010 年的 8.05/10 万上升到 2019 年的 10.86/10 万，年均变化百分比为 2.79%（P = 0.003）。北京市前列腺癌世标死亡率 2010 年为 3.08/10 万，2019 年为 3.20/10 万，年均变化百分比为 1.10%（P = 0.132）。

前列腺癌年龄别发病率和死亡率在 55 岁以前均较低，从 55 岁开始呈上升趋势，60 岁之后快速上升。城区和郊区发病率分别在 75~79 岁组和 80~84 岁组达到高峰，而死亡率均在 85 岁及以上年龄组达到高峰（图 5.16.1 至图 5.16.6）。

The ASR World for incidence of prostate cancer increased from 8.05 per 100,000 in 2010 to 10.86 per 100,000 in 2019; and the APC of ASR World for incidence was 2.79%（P = 0.003）. The ASR World for mortality was 3.08 per 100,000 in 2010 and 3.20 per 100,000 in 2019; and the APC of ASR World for mortality was 1.10%（P = 0.132）.

The age-specific incidence and mortality rates of prostate cancer were relatively low in males under 55 years old and increased constantly thereafter. The age-specific incidence and mortality rates increased dramatically in males older than 60 years old. The incidence rates peaked at the age groups of 75-79 years in urban areas and 80-84 years in peri-urban areas, respectively. The mortality rates in both urban and peri-urban areas peaked at the age group of 85 years and above（Figure 5.16.1-5.16.6）.

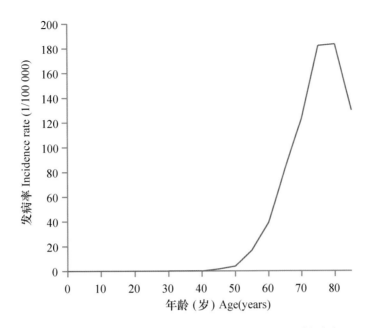

图 5.16.1 2019 年北京市户籍居民前列腺癌年龄别发病率
Figure 5.16.1 Age-specific incidence rates of prostate cancer in Beijing, 2019

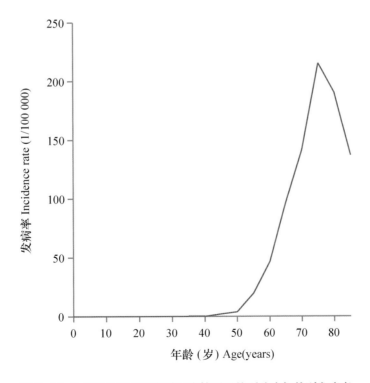

图 5.16.2 2019 年北京市城区户籍居民前列腺癌年龄别发病率
Figure 5.16.2 Age-specific incidence rates of prostate cancer in urban areas of Beijing, 2019

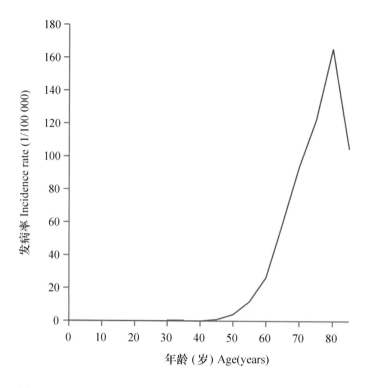

图 5.16.3 2019 年北京市郊区户籍居民前列腺癌年龄别发病率
Figure 5.16.3 Age-specific incidence rates of prostate cancer in peri-urban areas of Beijing, 2019

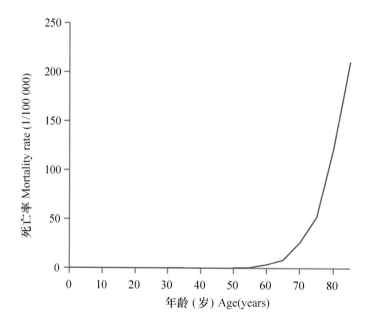

图 5.16.4 2019 年北京市户籍居民前列腺癌年龄别死亡率
Figure 5.16.4 Age-specific mortality rates of prostate cancer in Beijing, 2019

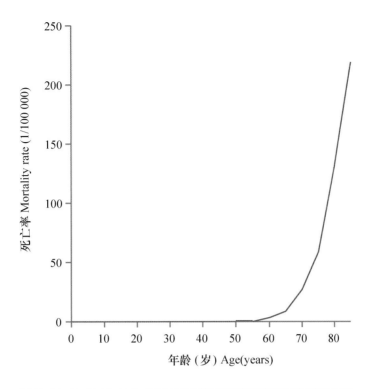

图 5.16.5 2019 年北京市城区户籍居民前列腺癌年龄别死亡率
Figure 5.16.5 Age-specific mortality rates of prostate cancer in urban areas of Beijing, 2019

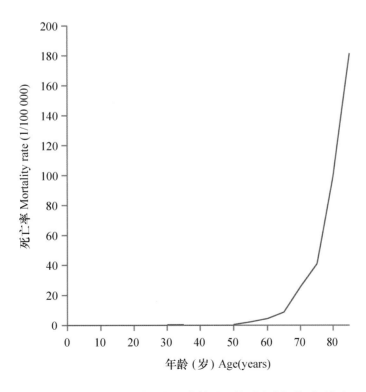

图 5.16.6 2019 年北京市郊区户籍居民前列腺癌年龄别死亡率
Figure 5.16.6 Age-specific mortality rates of prostate cancer in peri-urban areas of Beijing, 2019

2019 年，北京市前列腺癌世标发病率和死亡率在 16 个辖区间有一定差异，城区发病率和死亡率均高于郊区（图 5.16.7 和图 5.16.8）。

In 2019, there were some differences among the 16 districts in ASR World for incidence and mortality of prostate cancer in Beijing. The incidence and mortality rates were both higher in urban areas than in peri-urban areas（Figure 5.16.7-5.16.8）.

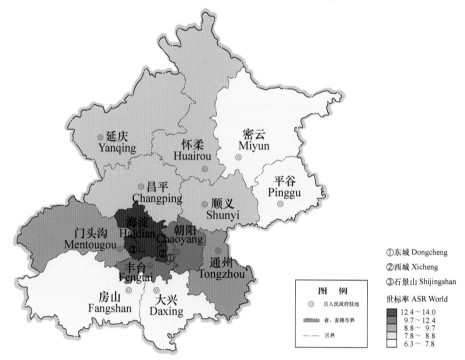

图 5.16.7 2019 年北京市户籍居民前列腺癌世标发病率（1/10⁵）地区分布情况
Figure 5.16.7 ASRs World for incidence of prostate cancer（$1/10^5$）by district in Beijing, 2019

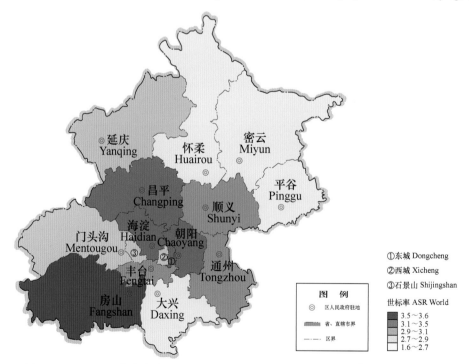

图 5.16.8 2019 年北京市户籍居民前列腺癌世标死亡率（1/10⁵）地区分布情况
Figure 5.16.8 ASRs World for mortality of prostate cancer（$1/10^5$）by district in Beijing, 2019

（撰稿 李慧超，校稿 刘硕）

5.17 肾及泌尿系统部位不明（C64–66, C68）

5.17 Kidney & unspecified urinary organs（C64–66, C68）

2019 年，北京市肾及泌尿系统部位不明癌新发病例数为 2 379 例，占全部恶性肿瘤发病的 4.09%，位居恶性肿瘤发病第 7 位；其中男性 1 504 例，女性 875 例，城区 1 628 例，郊区 751 例。肾及泌尿系统部位不明癌发病率为 17.16/10 万，中标发病率为 8.78/10 万，世标发病率为 8.60/10 万；男性世标发病率为女性的 2.02 倍，城区世标发病率为郊区的 1.18 倍。0~74 岁累积发病率为 1.00%（表 5.17.1）。

There were 2,379 new cases diagnosed as cancer of kidney & unspecified urinary organs（1,504 males and 875 females, 1,628 in urban areas and 751 in peri-urban areas）, accounting for 4.09% of new cases of all cancers in 2019. Cancer of kidney & unspecified urinary organs was the 7th common cancer in Beijing. The crude incidence rate was 17.16 per 100,000, with an ASR China and an ASR World of 8.78 and 8.60 per 100,000, respectively. The ASR World for incidence was 102% higher in males than in females and 18% higher in urban areas than in peri-urban areas. The cumulative incidence rate for subjects aged 0 to 74 years was 1.00%（Table 5.17.1）.

表 5.17.1 2019 年北京市户籍居民肾及泌尿系统部位不明癌发病情况
Table 5.17.1 Incidence of cancer of kidney & unspecified urinary organs in Beijing, 2019

地区 Area	性别 Sex	例数 No. of cases	粗率 Crude rate （1/10⁵）	构成比 Freq.（%）	中标率 ASR China （1/10⁵）	世标率 ASR World （1/10⁵）	累积率 Cumulative rate（0~74, %）	顺位 Rank
全市 All areas	合计 Both	2 379	17.16	4.09	8.78	8.60	1.00	7
	男性 Male	1 504	21.81	5.26	11.71	11.55	1.36	7
	女性 Female	875	12.55	2.95	5.91	5.72	0.64	6
城区 Urban areas	合计 Both	1 628	19.06	4.28	9.36	9.10	1.06	6
	男性 Male	1 017	23.98	5.50	12.43	12.11	1.45	7
	女性 Female	611	14.20	3.12	6.37	6.16	0.68	6
郊区 Peri-urban areas	合计 Both	751	14.11	3.72	7.76	7.69	0.89	7
	男性 Male	487	18.36	4.83	10.48	10.50	1.23	7
	女性 Female	264	9.89	2.62	5.11	4.95	0.58	7

2019年，北京市肾及泌尿系统部位不明癌死亡病例数为775例，占全部恶性肿瘤死亡的2.83%，位居恶性肿瘤死亡第11位；其中男性464例，女性311例，城区570例，郊区205例。肾及泌尿系统部位不明癌死亡率为5.59/10万，中标死亡率为2.05/10万，世标死亡率为2.07/10万；男性世标死亡率为女性的1.97倍，城区世标死亡率为郊区的1.29倍。0~74岁累积死亡率为0.20%（表5.17.2）。

A total of 775 cases died of cancer of kidney & unspecified urinary organs（464 males and 311 females, 570 in urban areas and 205 in peri-urban areas）, accounting for 2.83% of all cancer deaths in 2019. Cancer of kidney & unspecified urinary organs was the 11th leading cause of cancer deaths in all cancers. The crude mortality rate was 5.59 per 100,000, with an ASR China and an ASR World of 2.05 and 2.07 per 100,000, respectively. The ASR World for mortality was 97% higher in males than in females and 29% higher in urban areas than in peri-urban areas. The cumulative mortality rate for subjects aged 0 to 74 years was 0.20%（Table 5.17.2）.

表5.17.2 2019年北京市户籍居民肾及泌尿系统部位不明癌死亡情况
Table 5.17.2 Mortality of cancer of kidney & unspecified urinary organs in Beijing, 2019

地区 Area	性别 Sex	例数 No. of deaths	粗率 Crude rate （1/10⁵）	构成比 Freq.（%）	中标率 ASR China （1/10⁵）	世标率 ASR World （1/10⁵）	累积率 Cumulative rate（0~74, %）	顺位 Rank
全市 All areas	合计 Both	775	5.59	2.83	2.05	2.07	0.20	11
	男性 Male	464	6.73	2.86	2.73	2.78	0.29	12
	女性 Female	311	4.46	2.79	1.41	1.41	0.12	11
城区 Urban areas	合计 Both	570	6.67	3.19	2.22	2.24	0.22	10
	男性 Male	341	8.04	3.29	3.02	3.05	0.33	11
	女性 Female	229	5.32	3.06	1.46	1.47	0.13	10
郊区 Peri-urban areas	合计 Both	205	3.85	2.16	1.71	1.74	0.16	13
	男性 Male	123	4.64	2.11	2.20	2.27	0.23	12
	女性 Female	82	3.07	2.24	1.26	1.24	0.10	14

按部位划分，肾癌（C64）发病率为12.45/10万，中标发病率为6.88/10万，世标发病率为6.72/10万；肾癌死亡率为3.35/10万，中标死亡率为1.33/10万，世标死亡率为1.34/10万。肾盂癌（C65）发病率为2.08/10万，中标发病率为0.86/10万，世标发病率为0.85/10万；肾盂癌死亡率为0.89/10万，中标死亡率为0.27/10万，世标死亡率为0.28/10万。输尿管癌（C66）发病率为2.28/10万，中标发病率为0.91/10万，世标发病率为0.89/10万；输尿管癌死亡率为1.11/10万，中标死亡率和世标死亡率均为0.37/10万（表5.17.3至表5.17.8）。

By subsite, the kidney cancer（C64）incidence rate was 12.45 per 100,000, with an ASR China of 6.88 per 100,000 and an ASR World of 6.72 per 100,000; and the mortality rate was 3.35 per 100,000, with an ASR China of 1.33 per 100,000 and an ASR World of 1.34 per 100,000. The incidence rate of renal pelvis cancer（C65）was 2.08 per 100,000, with an ASR China of 0.86 per 100,000 and an ASR World of 0.85 per 100,000; and the mortality rate was 0.89 per 100,000, with an ASR China of 0.27 per 100,000 and an ASR World of 0.28 per 100,000. The ureter cancer（C66）incidence rate was 2.28 per 100,000, with an ASR China of 0.91 per 100,000 and an ASR World of 0.89 per 100,000; and the mortality rate was 1.11 per 100,000, with both ASR China and ASR World of 0.37 per 100,000（Table 5.17.3-5.17.8）.

表5.17.3 2019年北京市户籍居民肾癌（C64）发病情况
Table 5.17.3 Incidence of kidney cancer （C64） in Beijing, 2019

地区 Area	性别 Sex	例数 No. of cases	粗率 Crude rate （1/10^5）	构成比 Freq.（%）	中标率 ASR China （1/10^5）	世标率 ASR World （1/10^5）	累积率 Cumulative rate（0~74, %）
全市 All areas	合计 Both	1 726	12.45	2.96	6.88	6.72	0.78
	男性 Male	1 183	17.16	4.14	9.69	9.52	1.11
	女性 Female	543	7.79	1.83	4.15	4.00	0.46
城区 Urban areas	合计 Both	1 189	13.92	3.12	7.44	7.21	0.85
	男性 Male	809	19.07	4.37	10.42	10.11	1.21
	女性 Female	380	8.83	1.94	4.55	4.40	0.50
郊区 Peri-urban areas	合计 Both	537	10.09	2.66	5.93	5.89	0.66
	男性 Male	374	14.10	3.71	8.45	8.46	0.95
	女性 Female	163	6.10	1.62	3.48	3.37	0.38

表 5.17.4 2019 年北京市户籍居民肾癌（C64）死亡情况
Table 5.17.4 Mortality of kidney cancer （C64） in Beijing, 2019

地区 Area	性别 Sex	例数 No. of deaths	粗率 Crude rate （1/10^5）	构成比 Freq.（%）	中标率 ASR China （1/10^5）	世标率 ASR World （1/10^5）	累积率 Cumulative rate（0~74, %）
全市 All areas	合计 Both	464	3.35	1.70	1.33	1.34	0.15
	男性 Male	315	4.57	1.94	1.94	1.98	0.22
	女性 Female	149	2.14	1.34	0.76	0.75	0.08
城区 Urban areas	合计 Both	343	4.01	1.92	1.47	1.47	0.16
	男性 Male	237	5.59	2.29	2.22	2.23	0.25
	女性 Female	106	2.46	1.42	0.76	0.76	0.08
郊区 Peri-urban areas	合计 Both	121	2.27	1.27	1.05	1.09	0.12
	男性 Male	78	2.94	1.34	1.43	1.50	0.17
	女性 Female	43	1.61	1.17	0.71	0.71	0.08

表 5.17.5 2019 年北京市户籍居民肾盂癌（C65）发病情况
Table 5.17.5 Incidence of renal pelvis cancer （C65） in Beijing, 2019

地区 Area	性别 Sex	例数 No. of cases	粗率 Crude rate （1/10^5）	构成比 Freq.（%）	中标率 ASR China （1/10^5）	世标率 ASR World （1/10^5）	累积率 Cumulative rate（0~74, %）
全市 All areas	合计 Both	288	2.08	0.49	0.86	0.85	0.10
	男性 Male	139	2.02	0.49	0.90	0.90	0.12
	女性 Female	149	2.14	0.50	0.82	0.79	0.09
城区 Urban areas	合计 Both	192	2.25	0.50	0.86	0.85	0.10
	男性 Male	90	2.12	0.49	0.89	0.89	0.11
	女性 Female	102	2.37	0.52	0.83	0.80	0.09
郊区 Peri-urban areas	合计 Both	96	1.80	0.48	0.84	0.83	0.11
	男性 Male	49	1.85	0.49	0.89	0.91	0.13
	女性 Female	47	1.76	0.47	0.78	0.74	0.09

表 5.17.6 2019 年北京市户籍居民肾盂癌（C65）死亡情况
Table 5.17.6 Mortality of renal pelvis cancer （C65） in Beijing, 2019

地区 Area	性别 Sex	例数 No. of deaths	粗率 Crude rate （1/10⁵）	构成比 Freq.（%）	中标率 ASR China （1/10⁵）	世标率 ASR World （1/10⁵）	累积率 Cumulative rate(0~74, %)
全市 All areas	合计 Both	123	0.89	0.45	0.27	0.28	0.02
	男性 Male	58	0.84	0.36	0.31	0.32	0.03
	女性 Female	65	0.93	0.58	0.24	0.25	0.01
城区 Urban areas	合计 Both	95	1.11	0.53	0.30	0.31	0.02
	男性 Male	43	1.01	0.41	0.32	0.33	0.03
	女性 Female	52	1.21	0.70	0.28	0.29	0.02
郊区 Peri-urban areas	合计 Both	28	0.53	0.29	0.21	0.22	0.02
	男性 Male	15	0.57	0.26	0.27	0.27	0.02
	女性 Female	13	0.49	0.35	0.16	0.18	0.01

表 5.17.7 2019 年北京市户籍居民输尿管癌（C66）发病情况
Table 5.17.7 Incidence of ureter cancer （C66） in Beijing, 2019

地区 Area	性别 Sex	例数 No. of cases	粗率 Crude rate （1/10⁵）	构成比 Freq.（%）	中标率 ASR China （1/10⁵）	世标率 ASR World （1/10⁵）	累积率 Cumulative rate(0~74, %)
全市 All areas	合计 Both	316	2.28	0.54	0.91	0.89	0.10
	男性 Male	164	2.38	0.57	1.02	1.02	0.12
	女性 Female	152	2.18	0.51	0.80	0.77	0.08
城区 Urban areas	合计 Both	213	2.49	0.56	0.93	0.92	0.10
	男性 Male	106	2.50	0.57	1.02	1.02	0.12
	女性 Female	107	2.49	0.55	0.84	0.82	0.08
郊区 Peri-urban areas	合计 Both	103	1.93	0.51	0.86	0.85	0.11
	男性 Male	58	2.19	0.58	1.03	1.03	0.13
	女性 Female	45	1.69	0.45	0.71	0.69	0.08

表 5.17.8 2019 年北京市户籍居民输尿管癌（C66）死亡情况
Table 5.17.8 Mortality of ureter cancer （C66） in Beijing, 2019

地区 Area	性别 Sex	例数 No. of deaths	粗率 Crude rate （1/10⁵）	构成比 Freq.（%）	中标率 ASR China （1/10⁵）	世标率 ASR World （1/10⁵）	累积率 Cumulative rate（0~74，%）
全市 All areas	合计 Both	154	1.11	0.56	0.37	0.37	0.03
	男性 Male	79	1.15	0.49	0.44	0.43	0.04
	女性 Female	75	1.08	0.67	0.31	0.31	0.02
城区 Urban areas	合计 Both	105	1.23	0.59	0.37	0.37	0.04
	男性 Male	50	1.18	0.48	0.42	0.41	0.04
	女性 Female	55	1.28	0.74	0.32	0.33	0.03
郊区 Peri-urban areas	合计 Both	49	0.92	0.52	0.39	0.37	0.02
	男性 Male	29	1.09	0.50	0.49	0.48	0.03
	女性 Female	20	0.75	0.55	0.29	0.27	0.02

北京市肾及泌尿系统部位不明癌世标发病率由 2010 年的 6.72/10 万上升到 2019 年的 8.60/10 万，年均变化百分比为 2.42%（$P < 0.001$）；男性和女性世标发病率 10 年间年均变化百分比分别为 3.13%（$P < 0.001$）和 1.25%（$P = 0.060$）。北京市肾及泌尿系统部位不明癌世标死亡率 2010 年为 2.21/10 万，2019 年为 2.07/10 万，年均变化百分比为 -0.04%（$P = 0.964$）；男性和女性世标死亡率 10 年间年均变化百分比分别为 0.31%（$P = 0.805$）和 -0.55%（$P = 0.487$）。

肾及泌尿系统部位不明癌年龄别发病率在 30 岁之前均处于较低水平，自 30~34 岁组开始快速上升，至 80~84 岁组达到高峰；年龄别死亡率自 50~54 岁组开始快速上升。除 30~34 岁组死亡

The ASR World for incidence of cancer of kidney & unspecified urinary organs increased from 6.72 per 100,000 in 2010 to 8.60 per 100,000 in 2019; and the APC of ASR World for incidence was 2.42%（$P < 0.001$）. The APCs of ASR World for incidence of cancer of kidney & unspecified urinary organs in males and females were 3.13%（$P < 0.001$）and 1.25%（$P = 0.060$）, respectively. The ASR World for mortality of cancer of kidney & unspecified urinary organs was 2.21 per 100,000 in 2010 and 2.07 per 100,000 in 2019; and the APC of ASR World for mortality was − 0.04%（$P = 0.964$）. The APCs of ASR World for mortality of cancer of kidney & unspecified urinary organs in males and females were 0.31%（$P = 0.805$）and − 0.55%（$P = 0.487$）, respectively.

The age-specific incidence of cancer of kidney & unspecified urinary organs was at a low level in age below 30 years, and thereafter increased rapidly, peaking at the age group of 80-84 years. The age-specific mortality rate increased rapidly at the age group of 50-54 years. Except for the age group of 30-34 years of mortality, age-specific incidence and

率外，各年龄组男性发病率和死亡率均高于女性。城区和郊区年龄别发病率、死亡率变化有一定差异（图 5.17.1 至图 5.17.6）。

mortality rates in males were generally higher than those in females. There were some differences in age-specific incidence and mortality rates between urban and peri-urban areas（Figure 5.17.1-5.17.6）.

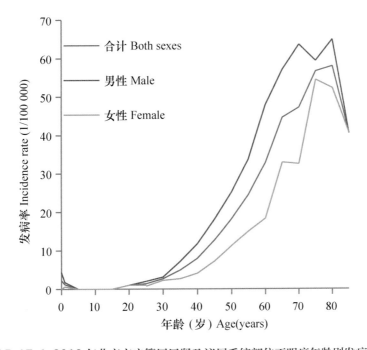

图 5.17.1 2019 年北京市户籍居民肾及泌尿系统部位不明癌年龄别发病率
Figure 5.17.1 Age-specific incidence rates of cancer of kidney & unspecified urinary organs in Beijing, 2019

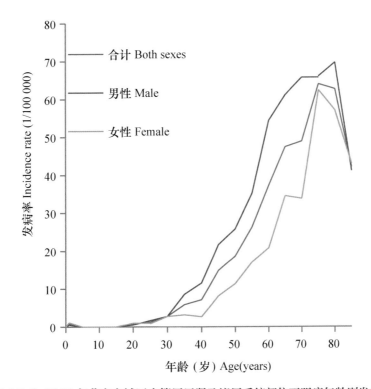

图 5.17.2 2019 年北京市城区户籍居民肾及泌尿系统部位不明癌年龄别发病率
Figure 5.17.2 Age-specific incidence rates of cancer of kidney & unspecified urinary organs in urban areas of Beijing, 2019

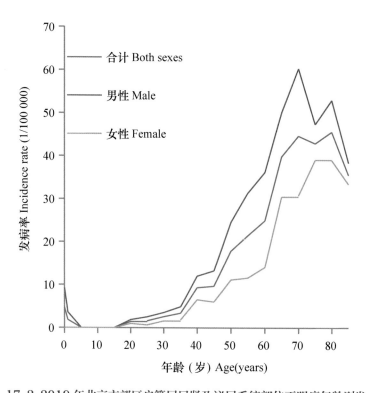

图 5.17.3 2019 年北京市郊区户籍居民肾及泌尿系统部位不明癌年龄别发病率
Figure 5.17.3 Age-specific incidence rates of cancer of kidney & unspecified urinary organs in peri-urban areas of Beijing, 2019

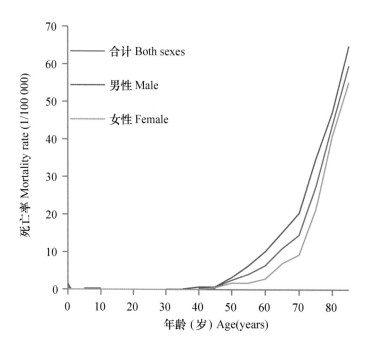

图 5.17.4 2019 年北京市户籍居民肾及泌尿系统部位不明癌年龄别死亡率
Figure 5.17.4 Age-specific mortality rates of cancer of kidney & unspecified urinary organs in Beijing, 2019

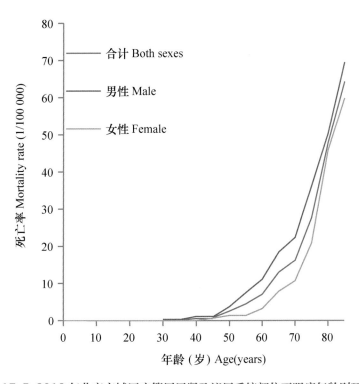

图 5.17.5 2019 年北京市城区户籍居民肾及泌尿系统部位不明癌年龄别死亡率
Figure 5.17.5 Age-specific mortality rates of cancer of kidney & unspecified urinary organs in urban areas of Beijing, 2019

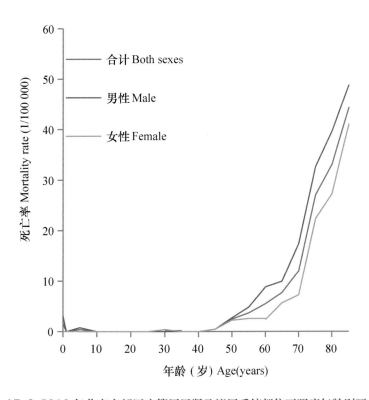

图 5.17.6 2019 年北京市郊区户籍居民肾及泌尿系统部位不明癌年龄别死亡率
Figure 5.17.6 Age-specific mortality rates of cancer of kidney & unspecified urinary organs in peri-urban areas of Beijing, 2019

2019年，北京市肾及泌尿系统部位不明癌世标发病率和死亡率在16个辖区间有一定差异，城区发病率和死亡率均高于郊区（图5.17.7和图5.17.8）。

In 2019, there were some differences among the 16 districts in ASR World for incidence and mortality of cancer of kidney & unspecified urinary organs in Beijing. The incidence and mortality rates were higher in urban areas than in peri-urban areas（Figure 5.17.7-5.17.8）.

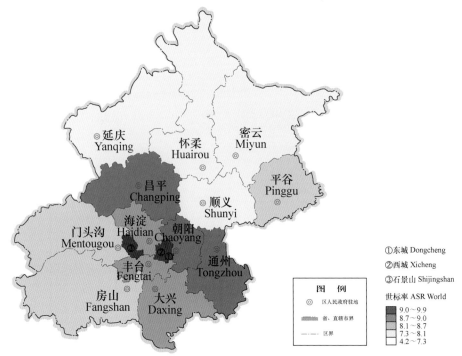

图5.17.7 2019年北京市户籍居民肾及泌尿系统部位不明癌世标发病率（1/10^5）地区分布情况
Figure 5.17.7 ASRs World for incidence of cancer of kidney & unspecified urinary organs（1/10^5）by district in Beijing, 2019

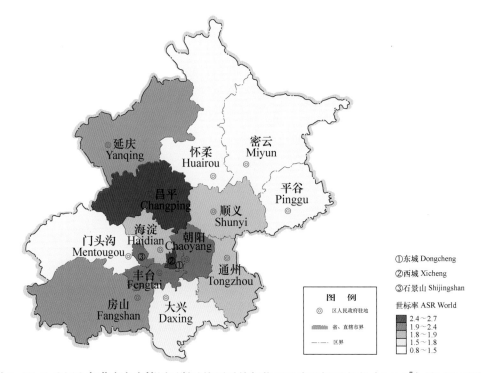

图5.17.8 2019年北京市户籍居民肾及泌尿系统部位不明癌世标死亡率（1/10^5）地区分布情况
Figure 5.17.8 ASRs World for mortality of cancer of kidney & unspecified urinary organs（1/10^5）by district in Beijing, 2019

肾（除外肾盂）是肾及泌尿系统部位不明癌发生的最主要的亚部位，占全部病例的72.55%。其后依次为肾盂、输尿管和其他泌尿器官，分别占12.11%、13.28%和2.06%（图5.17.9）。

Kidney（except renal pelvis）was the most common subsite of cancer of kidney & unspecified urinary organs, accounting for 72.55% of all cases, followed by the renal pelvis（12.11%）, the ureter（13.28%）, and the other urinary organs（2.06%）（Figure 5.17.9）.

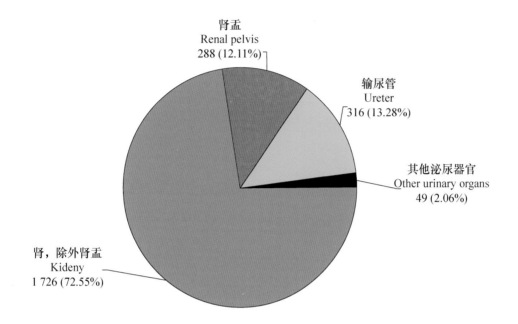

图5.17.9　2019年北京市户籍居民肾及泌尿系统部位不明癌亚部位分布情况
Figure 5.17.9 Subsite distribution of cancer of kidney & unspecified urinary organs in Beijing, 2019

（撰稿 李慧超，校稿 刘硕）

5.18 膀胱（C67）

2019 年，北京市膀胱癌新发病例数为 1 922 例，占全部恶性肿瘤发病的 3.30%，位居恶性肿瘤发病第 8 位；其中男性 1 473 例，女性 449 例，城区 1 291 例，郊区 631 例。膀胱癌发病率为 13.86/10 万，中标发病率为 5.86/10 万，世标发病率为 5.83/10 万；男性世标发病率为女性的 3.76 倍，城区世标发病率为郊区的 1.07 倍。0~74 岁累积发病率为 0.72%（表 5.18.1）。

5.18 Bladder（C67）

There were 1,922 new cases diagnosed as bladder cancer（1,473 males and 449 females, 1,291 in urban areas and 631 in peri-urban areas）, accounting for 3.30% of new cases of all cancers in 2019. Bladder cancer was the 8th common cancer in Beijing. The crude incidence rate was 13.86 per 100,000, with an ASR China and an ASR World of 5.86 and 5.83 per 100,000, respectively. The ASR World for incidence was 276% higher in males than in females and 7% higher in urban areas than in peri urban areas. The cumulative incidence rate for subjects aged 0 to 74 years was 0.72%（Table 5.18.1）.

表 5.18.1 2019 年北京市户籍居民膀胱癌发病情况
Table 5.18.1 Incidence of bladder cancer in Beijing, 2019

地区 Area	性别 Sex	例数 No. of cases	粗率 Crude rate （1/10^5）	构成比 Freq.（%）	中标率 ASR China （1/10^5）	世标率 ASR World （1/10^5）	累积率 Cumulative rate（0~74, %）	顺位 Rank
全市 All areas	合计 Both	1 922	13.86	3.30	5.86	5.83	0.72	8
	男性 Male	1 473	21.36	5.16	9.45	9.42	1.16	8
	女性 Female	449	6.44	1.51	2.57	2.51	0.30	15
城区 Urban areas	合计 Both	1 291	15.11	3.39	6.02	5.97	0.73	9
	男性 Male	970	22.87	5.24	9.49	9.45	1.15	8
	女性 Female	321	7.46	1.64	2.80	2.74	0.33	15
郊区 Peri-urban areas	合计 Both	631	11.85	3.13	5.60	5.56	0.69	8
	男性 Male	503	18.96	4.99	9.36	9.37	1.17	6
	女性 Female	128	4.79	1.27	2.16	2.10	0.25	15

2019 年，北京市膀胱癌死亡病例数为 757 例，占全部恶性肿瘤死亡的 2.77%，位居恶性肿瘤死亡第 12 位；其中男性 570 例，女性 187 例，

A total of 757 cases died of bladder cancer（570 males and 187 females, 522 in urban areas and 235 in peri-urban areas）, accounting for 2.77% of all cancer deaths in 2019. Bladder cancer was the 12th leading cause of cancer deaths in all cancers. The

城区 522 例，郊区 235 例。膀胱癌死亡率为 5.46/10 万，中标死亡率为 1.71/10 万，世标死亡率为 1.75/10 万；男性世标死亡率为女性的 3.34 倍，郊区世标死亡率为城区的 1.02 倍。0~74 岁累积死亡率为 0.15%（表 5.18.2）。

crude mortality rate was 5.46 per 100,000, with an ASR China and an ASR World of 1.71 and 1.75 per 100,000, respectively. The ASR World for mortality was 234% higher in males than in females and 2% higher in peri-urban areas than in urban areas. The cumulative mortality rate for subjects aged 0 to 74 years was 0.15%（Table 5.18.2）.

表 5.18.2　2019 年北京市户籍居民膀胱癌死亡情况
Table 5.18.2 Mortality of bladder cancer in Beijing, 2019

地区 Area	性别 Sex	例数 No. of deaths	粗率 Crude rate （1/10⁵）	构成比 Freq.（%）	中标率 ASR China （1/10⁵）	世标率 ASR World （1/10⁵）	累积率 Cumulative rate（0~74, %）	顺位 Rank
全市 All areas	合计 Both	757	5.46	2.77	1.71	1.75	0.15	12
	男性 Male	570	8.27	3.52	2.73	2.81	0.23	10
	女性 Female	187	2.68	1.68	0.83	0.84	0.08	16
城区 Urban areas	合计 Both	522	6.11	2.92	1.69	1.74	0.14	12
	男性 Male	385	9.08	3.71	2.63	2.72	0.22	10
	女性 Female	137	3.19	1.83	0.87	0.88	0.07	15
郊区 Peri-urban areas	合计 Both	235	4.41	2.47	1.77	1.77	0.16	11
	男性 Male	185	6.97	3.17	2.96	2.99	0.24	9
	女性 Female	50	1.87	1.36	0.74	0.74	0.08	16

北京市膀胱癌世标发病率由 2010 年的 5.27/10 万上升到 2019 年的 5.83/10 万，年均变化百分比为 0.94%（$P = 0.010$）；男性和女性世标发病率 10 年间年均变化百分比分别为 1.22%（$P = 0.008$）和 0.23%（$P = 0.779$）。北京市膀胱癌世标死亡率 2010 年为 1.86/10 万，2019 年为 1.75/10 万，年均变化百分比为 0.07%（$P =$

The ASR World for incidence of bladder cancer increased from 5.27 per 100,000 in 2010 to 5.83 per 100,000 in 2019; and the APC of ASR World for incidence was 0.94%（$P = 0.010$）.The APCs of ASR World for incidence of bladder cancer in males and females were 1.22%（$P = 0.008$）and 0.23%（$P = 0.779$）, respectively. The ASR World for mortality of bladder cancer was 1.86 per 100,000 in 2010 and 1.75 per 100,000 in 2019; and the APC of ASR World for mortality was 0.07%（$P = 0.925$）. The APCs of ASR World for

0.925）；男性和女性世标死亡率 10 年间年均变化百分比分别为 0.44%（*P*=0.623）和 −0.42%（*P*=0.697）。

膀胱癌年龄别发病率和死亡率呈现明显的性别差异。男性和女性发病率均自 50～54 岁组开始快速上升，至 80～84 岁组达到高峰（125.38/10 万和 38.83/10 万）。男性和女性死亡率均自 65～69 岁组开始快速上升，至 85 岁及以上年龄组达到高峰（152.00/10 万 和 42.52/10 万）。除 40 岁以下年龄组略有波动外，男性发病率和死亡率均高于女性。城区和郊区年龄别发病率、死亡率变化有一定差异，但总体趋势相同（图 5.18.1 至图 5.18.6）。

mortality of bladder cancer in males and females were 0.44%（*P*=0.623）and −0.42%（*P*=0.697）, respectively.

The trends of age-specific incidence and mortality rates showed differences between males and females in Beijing. The incidence rates in males and in females both increased rapidly from the age group of 50-54 years and peaked at the age group of 80-84 years（125.38 per 100,000 and 38.83 per 100,000, respectively）. The mortality rates in males and in females both increased significantly from the age group of 65-69 years and peaked at the age group of 85 years and above（152.00 per 100,000 and 42.52 per 100,000, respectively）. Except for some fluctuations before 40 years old, the age-specific incidence and mortality rates in males were consistently higher than those in females. There were some differences in age-specific incidence and mortality rates between urban and peri-urban areas, but the overall trends were same（Figure 5.18.1-5.18.6）.

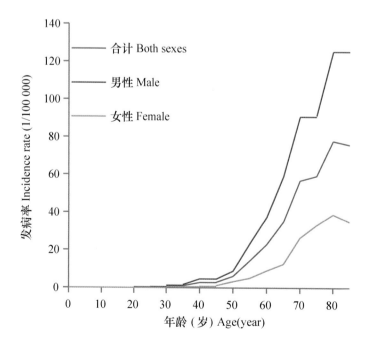

图 5.18.1 2019 年北京市户籍居民膀胱癌年龄别发病率
Figure 5.18.1 Age-specific incidence rates of bladder cancer in Beijing, 2019

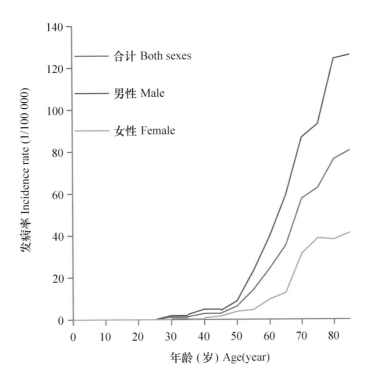

图 5.18.2 2019 年北京市城区户籍居民膀胱癌年龄别发病率

Figure 5.18.2 Age-specific incidence rates of bladder cancer in urban areas of Beijing, 2019

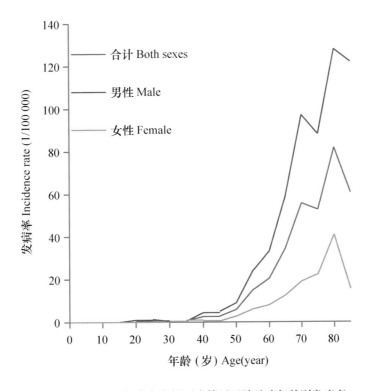

图 5.18.3 2019 年北京市郊区户籍居民膀胱癌年龄别发病率

Figure 5.18.3 Age-specific incidence rates of bladder cancer in peri-urban areas of Beijing, 2019

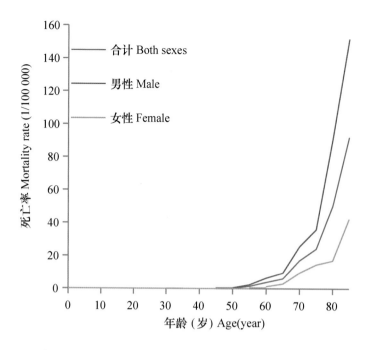

图 5.18.4 2019 年北京市户籍居民膀胱癌年龄别死亡率
Figure 5.18.4 Age-specific mortality rates of bladder cancer in Beijing, 2019

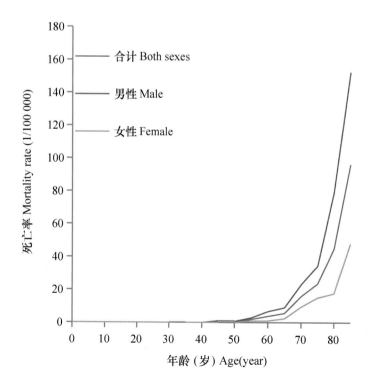

图 5.18.5 2019 年北京市城区户籍居民膀胱癌年龄别死亡率
Figure 5.18.5 Age-specific mortality rates of bladder cancer in urban areas of Beijing, 2019

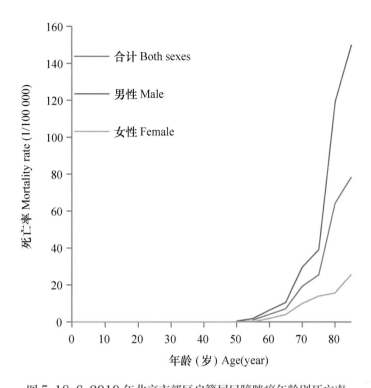

图 5.18.6 2019 年北京市郊区户籍居民膀胱癌年龄别死亡率
Figure 5.18.6 Age-specific mortality rates of bladder cancer in peri-urban areas of Beijing, 2019

2019 年，北京市膀胱癌世标发病率和死亡率在 16 个辖区间有一定差异，城区发病率高于郊区，郊区死亡率高于城区（图 5.18.7 和图 5.18.8）。

In 2019, there were some differences among the 16 districts in ASR World for incidence and mortality of bladder cancer in Beijing. The incidence rate was higher in urban areas than in peri-urban areas while the mortality rate was higher in peri-urban areas than in urban areas（Figure 5.18.7-5.18.8）.

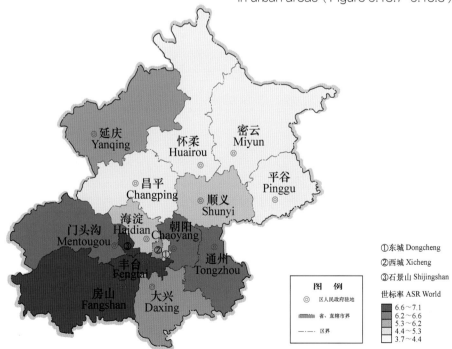

图 5.18.7 2019 年北京市户籍居民膀胱癌世标发病率（1/10^5）地区分布情况
Figure 5.18.7 ASRs World for incidence of bladder cancer（1/10^5）by district in Beijing, 2019

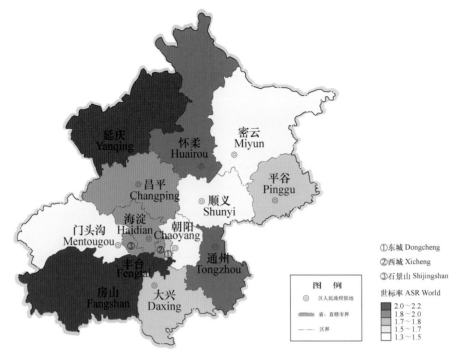

图 5.18.8 2019 年北京市户籍居民膀胱癌世标死亡率（1/10^5）地区分布情况
Figure 5.18.8 ASRs World for mortality of bladder cancer（1/10^5）by district in Beijing, 2019

全部膀胱癌新发病例中，有明确亚部位的病例占 40.48%。其中膀胱侧壁占 51.93%，膀胱后壁占 16.07%，膀胱前壁占 7.71%，输尿管口占 6.55%，膀胱三角区占 5.78%，膀胱顶和膀胱颈均占 5.53%，脐尿管占 0.64%，交搭跨越占 0.26%（图 5.18.9）。

About 40.48% cases were assigned to specified categories of bladder cancer site. Among those, 51.93% of cases occurred in the lateral wall of bladder, followed by the posterior wall of bladder（16.07%）, the anterior wall of bladder（7.71%）, the ureteric orifice（6.55%）,the trigone（5.78%）, the dome and the bladder neck（both of 5.53%）, the urachus（0.64%）and the overlapping（0.26%）（Figure 5.18.9）.

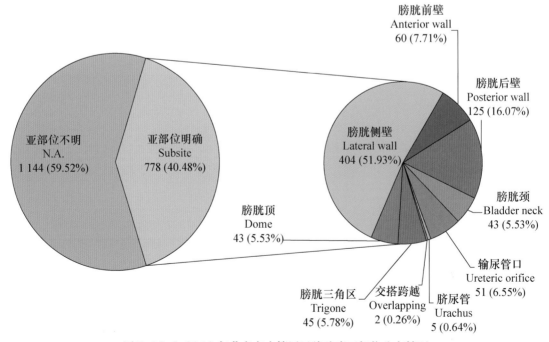

图 5.18.9 2019 年北京市户籍居民膀胱癌亚部位分布情况
Figure 5.18.9 Subsite distribution of bladder cancer in Beijing, 2019

（撰稿 李慧超，校稿 刘硕）

5.19 脑（C70-72）

2019 年，北京市脑癌新发病例数为 794 例，占全部恶性肿瘤发病的 1.36%，位居恶性肿瘤发病第 17 位；其中男性 438 例，女性 356 例，城区 522 例，郊区 272 例。脑癌发病率为 5.73/10 万，中标发病率为 4.08/10 万，世标发病率为 4.05/10 万；男性世标发病率为女性的 1.19 倍，城区世标发病率为郊区的 1.23 倍。0～74 岁累积发病率为 0.36%（表 5.19.1）。

5.19 Brain（C70-72）

There were 794 new cases diagnosed as brain cancer（438 males and 356 females, 522 in urban areas and 272 in peri-urban areas）, accounting for 1.36% of new cases of all cancers in 2019. Brain cancer was the 17th common cancer in Beijing. The crude incidence rate was 5.73 per 100,000, with an ASR China and an ASR World of 4.08 and 4.05 per 100,000, respectively. The ASR World for incidence was 19% higher in males than in females and 23% higher in urban areas than in peri-urban areas. The cumulative incidence rate for subjects aged 0 to 74 years was 0.36%（Table 5.19.1）.

表 5.19.1 2019 年北京市户籍居民脑癌发病情况
Table 5.19.1 Incidence of brain cancer in Beijing, 2019

地区 Area	性别 Sex	例数 No. of cases	粗率 Crude rate （1/10^5）	构成比 Freq.（%）	中标率 ASR China （1/10^5）	世标率 ASR World （1/10^5）	累积率 Cumulative rate（0~74, %）	顺位 Rank
全市 All areas	合计 Both	794	5.73	1.36	4.08	4.05	0.36	17
	男性 Male	438	6.35	1.53	4.50	4.41	0.41	15
	女性 Female	356	5.11	1.20	3.68	3.70	0.31	16
城区 Urban areas	合计 Both	522	6.11	1.37	4.41	4.38	0.38	18
	男性 Male	281	6.62	1.52	4.69	4.54	0.42	15
	女性 Female	241	5.60	1.23	4.16	4.25	0.35	16
郊区 Peri-urban areas	合计 Both	272	5.11	1.35	3.59	3.55	0.33	17
	男性 Male	157	5.92	1.56	4.23	4.24	0.40	15
	女性 Female	115	4.31	1.14	2.96	2.88	0.26	17

2019 年，北京市脑癌死亡病例数为 571 例，占全部恶性肿瘤死亡的 2.09%，位居恶性肿瘤死亡第 14 位；其中男性 293 例，女性 278 例，城区 348 例，郊区 223 例。脑癌死亡率为 4.12/10 万，

A total of 571 cases died of brain cancer（293 males and 278 females, 348 in urban areas and 223 in peri-urban areas）, accounting for 2.09% of all cancer deaths in 2019. Brain cancer was the 14th leading cause of cancer deaths in all cancers. The crude mortality rate was 4.12 per 100,000, with both ASR

中标死亡率和世标死亡率均为 2.21/10 万；男性世标死亡率为女性的 1.17 倍，郊区世标死亡率为城区的 1.11 倍。0~74 岁累积死亡率为 0.23%（表5.19.2）。

China and ASR World of 2.21 per 100,000. The ASR World for mortality was 17% higher in males than in females and 11% higher in peri-urban areas than in urban areas. The cumulative mortality rate for subjects aged 0 to 74 years was 0.23%（Table 5.19.2）.

表 5.19.2 2019 年北京市户籍居民脑癌死亡情况
Table 5.19.2 Mortality of brain cancer in Beijing, 2019

地区 Area	性别 Sex	例数 No. of deaths	粗率 Crude rate（1/10^5）	构成比 Freq.（%）	中标率 ASR China（1/10^5）	世标率 ASR World（1/10^5）	累积率 Cumulative rate（0~74, %）	顺位 Rank
全市 All areas	合计 Both	571	4.12	2.09	2.21	2.21	0.23	14
	男性 Male	293	4.25	1.81	2.36	2.38	0.25	13
	女性 Female	278	3.99	2.49	2.07	2.03	0.21	12
城区 Urban areas	合计 Both	348	4.07	1.95	2.08	2.13	0.22	14
	男性 Male	185	4.36	1.78	2.18	2.31	0.24	13
	女性 Female	163	3.79	2.18	1.98	1.96	0.19	13
郊区 Peri-urban areas	合计 Both	223	4.19	2.35	2.46	2.36	0.24	12
	男性 Male	108	4.07	1.85	2.62	2.49	0.25	13
	女性 Female	115	4.31	3.14	2.27	2.22	0.23	11

北京市脑癌世标发病率 2010 年为 3.57/10 万，2019 年为 4.05/10 万，年均变化百分比为 0.23%（$P=0.756$）；男性和女性标化发病率 10 年间年均变化百分比分别为 0.40%（$P=0.611$）和 0.03%（$P=0.978$）。北京市脑癌世标死亡率 2010 年为 2.25/10 万，2019 年为 2.21/10 万，年均变化百分比为 −0.71%（$P=0.446$）；男性和女性世标死

The ASR World for incidence of brain cancer was 3.57 per 100,000 in 2010 and 4.05 per 100,000 in 2019; and the APC of ASR World for incidence was 0.23%（$P=0.756$）. The APCs of ASR World for incidence of brain cancer in males and females were 0.40%（$P=0.611$）and 0.03%（$P=0.978$）, respectively. The ASR World for mortality of brain cancer was 2.25 per 100,000 in 2010 and 2.21 per 100,000 in 2019; and the APC of ASR World for mortality was −0.71%（$P=0.446$）. The APCs of ASR World for mortality of brain

亡率 10 年间年均变化百分比分别为 - 0.73% (*P* = 0.544) 和 - 0.64% (*P* = 0.570)。

脑癌年龄别发病率和死亡率在 5~9 岁组较高，10 岁后略有波动，40 岁以后快速上升（图 5.19.1 至图 5.19.6）。男性和女性的发病率分别在 80~84 岁组和 85 岁及以上年龄组达到高峰，死亡率均在 80~84 岁组达到高峰；除 75~79 岁年龄组外，50~54 岁及以上各年龄组男性发病率均高于女性（图 5.19.1 和图 5.19.4）。城区和郊区年龄别发病率、死亡率变化有一定差异，但总体趋势相同（图 5.19.2 和图 5.19.3，图 5.19.5 和图 5.19.6）。

cancer in males and females were - 0.73% (*P* = 0.544) and - 0.64% (*P* = 0.570) , respectively.

The age-specific incidence and mortality rates of brain cancer were relatively high at the age group of 5~9 years, and slight fluctuation were observed since 10 years old. The rates increased sharply in people older than 40 years old (Figure 5.19.1-5.19.6) . The age-specific incidence rates in males and females peaked at the age group of 80-84 years and 85 years and above, respectively, while the age-specific mortality rates peaked at the age group of 80-84 years for both sexes. Except for the age group of 75-79 years old, the age-specific incidence and mortality rates of brain cancer were consistently higher in males than in females starting from the age group of 50-54 (Figure 5.19.1, Figure 5.19.4) . There were some differences in age-specific incidence and mortality rates between urban and peri-urban areas, but the overall trends were same (Figure 5.19.2-5.19.3, Figure 5.19.5-5.19.6) .

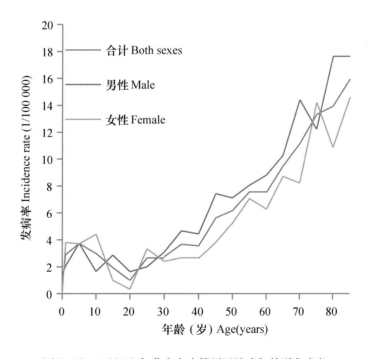

图 5.19.1 2019 年北京市户籍居民脑癌年龄别发病率
Figure 5.19.1 Age-specific incidence rates of brain cancer in Beijing, 2019

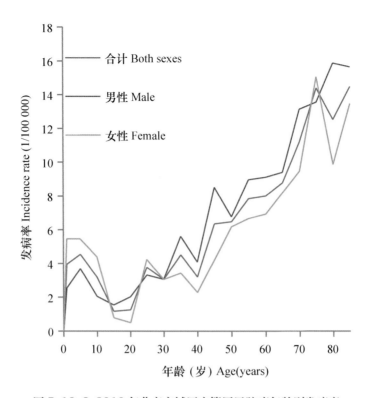

图 5.19.2 2019 年北京市城区户籍居民脑癌年龄别发病率
Figure 5.19.2 Age-specific incidence rates of brain cancer in urban areas of Beijing, 2019

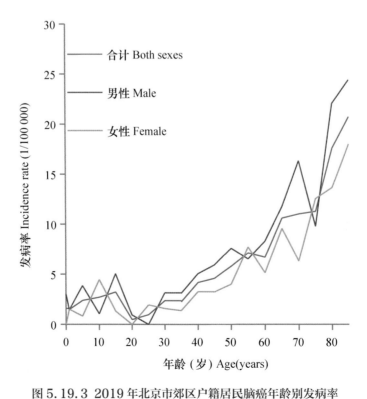

图 5.19.3 2019 年北京市郊区户籍居民脑癌年龄别发病率
Figure 5.19.3 Age-specific incidence rates of brain cancer in peri-urban areas of Beijing, 2019

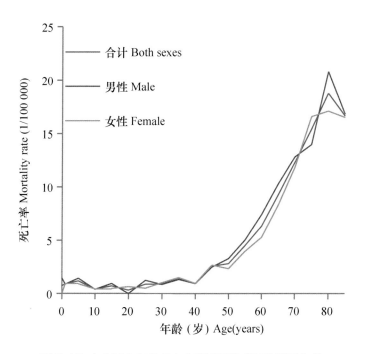

图 5.19.4 2019 年北京市户籍居民脑癌年龄别死亡率
Figure 5.19.4 Age-specific mortality rates of brain cancer in Beijing, 2019

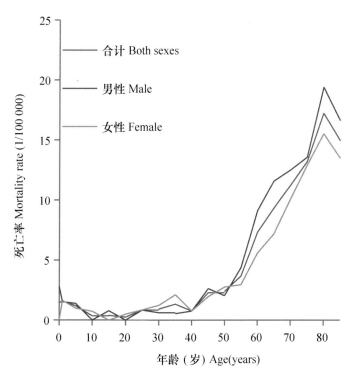

图 5.19.5 2019 年北京市城区户籍居民脑癌年龄别死亡率
Figure 5.19.5 Age-specific mortality rates of brain cancer in urban areas of Beijing, 2019

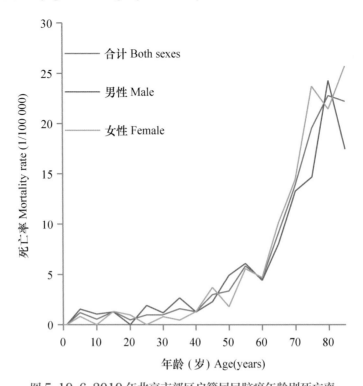

图 5.19.6 2019 年北京市郊区户籍居民脑癌年龄别死亡率
Figure 5.19.6 Age-specific mortality rates of brain cancer in peri-urban areas of Beijing, 2019

全部脑恶性肿瘤（C71）新发病例中，有明确亚部位的病例占 64.39%。其中额叶是最常见的发病部位，占 28.07%；其后依次为交搭跨越、颞叶和大脑（除外脑叶和脑室），分别占全部脑恶性肿瘤的 21.00%、17.88% 和 9.36%（图 5.19.7）。

About 64.39% cases were assigned to specified categories of brain cancer（C71）site. Among those, the frontal lobe was the most common site, accounting for 28.07% of all cases, followed by the overlapping part（21.00%），the temporal lobe（17.88%）and the cerebrum（except lobes and ventricles）（9.36%）（Figure 5.19.7）.

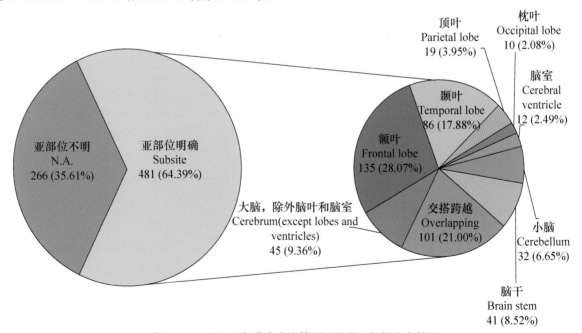

图 5.19.7 2019 年北京市户籍居民脑癌亚部位分布情况
Figure 5.19.7 Subsite distribution of brain cancer in Beijing, 2019

（撰稿 李晴雨，校稿 刘硕）

5.20 甲状腺（C73）

2019 年，北京市甲状腺癌新发病例数为 6 244 例，占全部恶性肿瘤发病的 10.72%，位居恶性肿瘤发病第 3 位；其中男性 1 799 例，女性 4 445 例，城区 3 947 例，郊区 2 297 例。甲状腺癌发病率为 45.03/10 万，中标发病率为 41.88/10 万，世标发病率为 34.75/10 万；女性世标发病率为男性的 2.43 倍，城区世标发病率是郊区的 1.11 倍。0~74 岁累积发病率为 3.05%（表 5.20.1）。

5.20 Thyroid（C73）

There were 6,244 new cases diagnosed as thyroid cancer（1,799 males and 4,445 females, 3,947 in urban areas and 2,297 in peri-urban areas）, accounting for 10.72% of all cancers in 2019. Thyroid cancer was the 3rd common cancer in Beijing. The crude incidence rate was 45.03 per 100,000, with an ASR China and an ASR World of 41.88 and 34.75 per 100,000, respectively. The ASR World for incidence was 143% higher in females than in males and 11% higher in urban areas than in peri-urban areas. The cumulative incidence rate for subjects aged 0 to 74 years was 3.05%（Table 5.20.1）.

表 5.20.1 2019 年北京市户籍居民甲状腺癌发病情况
Table 5.20.1 Incidence of thyroid cancer in Beijing, 2019

地区 Area	性别 Sex	例数 No. of cases	粗率 Crude rate （1/10^5）	构成比 Freq.（%）	中标率 ASR China （1/10^5）	世标率 ASR World （1/10^5）	累积率 Cumulative rate（0~74, %）	顺位 Rank
全市 All areas	合计 Both	6 244	45.03	10.72	41.88	34.75	3.05	3
	男性 Male	1 799	26.09	6.30	25.10	20.30	1.75	4
	女性 Female	4 445	63.76	14.98	58.73	49.27	4.36	3
城区 Urban areas	合计 Both	3 947	46.20	10.37	43.78	36.16	3.19	4
	男性 Male	1 191	28.08	6.44	27.49	22.15	1.91	5
	女性 Female	2 756	64.07	14.08	60.09	50.19	4.47	3
郊区 Peri-urban areas	合计 Both	2 297	43.15	11.39	38.97	32.57	2.84	3
	男性 Male	608	22.92	6.04	21.46	17.43	1.49	4
	女性 Female	1 689	63.25	16.74	56.68	47.86	4.19	3

2019 年，北京市甲状腺癌死亡病例数为 107 例，占全部恶性肿瘤死亡的 0.39%，位居恶性肿瘤死亡第 21 位；其中男性 32 例，女性 75 例，城区 69 例，郊区 38 例。甲状腺癌死亡率为 0.77/10 万，中标死亡率为 0.32/10 万，世标死亡率为 0.31/10 万；女性世标死亡率为男性的 1.84 倍，郊区世标死亡率为城区的 1.06 倍。0～74 岁累积死亡率为 0.03%（表 5.20.2）。

A total of 107 cases died of thyroid cancer（32 males and 75 females, 69 in urban areas and 38 in peri-urban areas）, accounting for 0.39% of all cancer deaths in 2019. Thyroid cancer was the 21st leading cause of cancer deaths in all cancers. The crude mortality rate was 0.77 per 100,000, with an ASR China and an ASR World of 0.32 and 0.31 per 100,000, respectively. The ASR World for mortality was 84% higher in females than in males and 6% higher in peri-urban areas than in urban areas. The cumulative mortality rate for subjects aged 0 to 74 years was 0.03%（Table 5.20.2）.

表 5.20.2 2019 年北京市户籍居民甲状腺癌死亡情况
Table 5.20.2 Mortality of thyroid cancer in Beijing, 2019

地区 Area	性别 Sex	例数 No. of deaths	粗率 Crude rate （1/10^5）	构成比 Freq.（%）	中标率 ASR China （1/10^5）	世标率 ASR World （1/10^5）	累积率 Cumulative rate（0~74, %）	顺位 Rank
全市 All areas	合计 Both	107	0.77	0.39	0.32	0.31	0.03	21
	男性 Male	32	0.46	0.20	0.22	0.21	0.03	20
	女性 Female	75	1.08	0.67	0.41	0.39	0.04	18
城区 Urban areas	合计 Both	69	0.81	0.39	0.31	0.30	0.03	21
	男性 Male	16	0.38	0.15	0.16	0.16	0.02	20
	女性 Female	53	1.23	0.71	0.45	0.44	0.05	18
郊区 Peri-urban areas	合计 Both	38	0.71	0.40	0.33	0.32	0.03	21
	男性 Male	16	0.60	0.27	0.32	0.31	0.03	19
	女性 Female	22	0.82	0.60	0.34	0.33	0.03	18

北京市甲状腺癌世标发病率由2010年的5.57/10万上升到2019年的34.75/10万，10年间年均变化百分比为20.86%（$P < 0.001$）；男性和女性10年间世标发病率年均变化百分比分别为23.71%（$P < 0.001$）和19.81%（$P < 0.001$）。北京市甲状腺癌世标死亡率由2010年的0.38/10万下降到2019年的0.31/10万，10年间年均变化百分比为 -2.56%（$P = 0.046$）；男性和女性10年间世标死亡率年均变化百分比分别为 -2.00%（$P = 0.051$）和 -2.98%（$P = 0.145$）。

甲状腺癌好发于25~59岁组人群，其发病率在0~19岁组较低，自15岁起快速增长，在35~39岁组达到高峰，随后逐渐下降；女性各年龄段发病率均高于男性（图5.20.1至图5.20.3）。甲状腺癌死亡率在45岁之前较低，之后逐渐上升，至80~84岁组达到高峰（图5.20.4至图5.20.6）。城区和郊区年龄别发病率、死亡率变化有一定差异，但总体趋势相同，波动均较为明显（图5.20.2和图5.20.3，图5.20.5和图5.20.6）。

The ASR World for incidence of thyroid cancer increased from 5.57 per 100,000 in 2010 to 34.75 per 100,000 in 2019; and the APC of ASR World for incidence was 20.86% （$P < 0.001$）. The APCs of ASR World for incidence of thyroid cancer in males and females were 23.71% （$P < 0.001$）and 19.81% （$P < 0.001$）, respectively. The ASR World for mortality of thyroid cancer decreased from 0.38 per 100,000 in 2010 to 0.31 per 100,000 in 2019; and the APC of ASR World for mortality was -2.56%（$P = 0.046$）. The APCs of ASR World for mortality of thyroid cancer in males and females were -2.00%（$P = 0.051$）and -2.98%（$P = 0.145$）, respectively.

Thyroid cancer was common at the age of 25-59 years old. The incidence rate was relatively low at the age group of 0-19 years old, and increased sharply thereafter, peaking at the age group of 40-44 years old, but started to go down gradually from age 45 onwards. The age-specific incidence rates were higher in females than in males at all age groups （Figure 5.20.1-5.20.3）. The mortality rate was relatively low before 45 years old, but increased gradually with slightly fluctuation thereafter, peaking at the age group of 80-84 years old（Figure 5.20.4-Figure 5.20.6）. There were some differences in age-specific incidence and mortality rates between urban and peri-urban areas, but the overall trends were same. The rates showed huge fluctuations （Figure 5.20.2-5.20.3, Figure 5.20.5-5.20.6）.

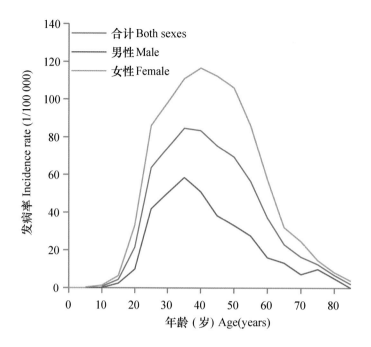

图 5.20.1 2019 年北京市户籍居民甲状腺癌年龄别发病率
Figure 5.20.1 Age-specific incidence rates of thyroid cancer in Beijing, 2019

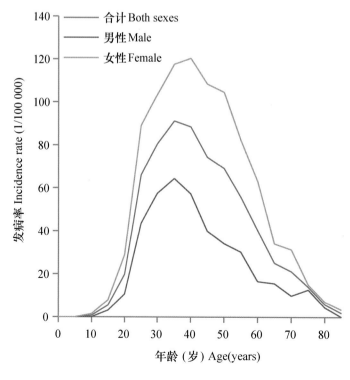

图 5.20.2 2019 年北京市城区户籍居民甲状腺癌年龄别发病率
Figure 5.20.2 Age-specific incidence rates of thyroid cancer in urban areas of Beijing, 2019

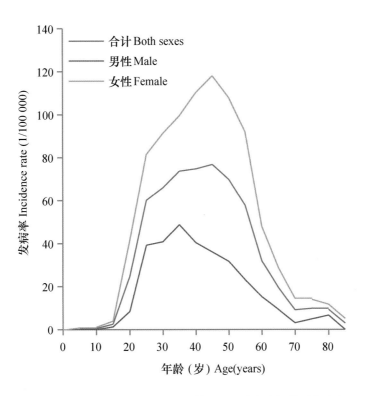

图 5.20.3　2019 年北京市郊区户籍居民甲状腺癌年龄别发病率

Figure 5.20.3 Age-specific incidence rates of thyroid cancer in peri-urban areas of Beijing, 2019

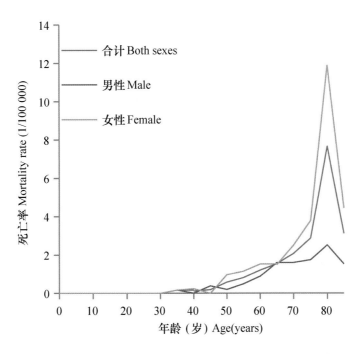

图 5.20.4　2019 年北京市户籍居民甲状腺癌年龄别死亡率

Figure 5.20.4 Age-specific mortality rates of thyroid cancer in Beijing, 2019

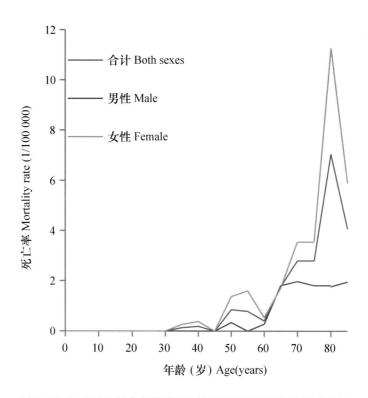

图 5.20.5 2019 年北京市城区户籍居民甲状腺癌年龄别死亡率
Figure 5.20.5 Age-specific mortality rates of thyroid cancer in urban areas of Beijing, 2019

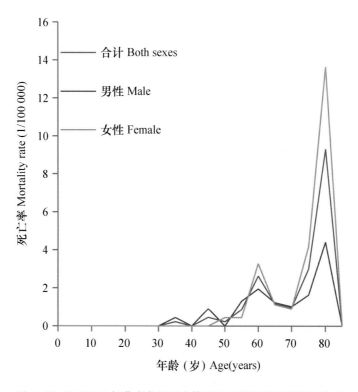

图 5.20.6 2019 年北京市郊区户籍居民甲状腺癌年龄别死亡率
Figure 5.20.6 Age-specific mortality rates of thyroid cancer in peri-urban areas of Beijing, 2019

2019 年，北京市甲状腺癌世标发病率在 16 个辖区间有显著差异，城区发病率高于郊区（图 5.20.7）。甲状腺癌世标死亡率在 16 个辖区间差异不明显（图 5.20.8）。

In 2019, there were significant differences among the 16 districts in ASR World for incidence of thyroid cancer in Beijing. The incidence rate was higher in urban areas than in peri-urban areas（Figure 5.20.7）. There was a slight difference among the 16 districts in ASR World for mortality of thyroid cancer in Beijing（Figure 5.20.8）.

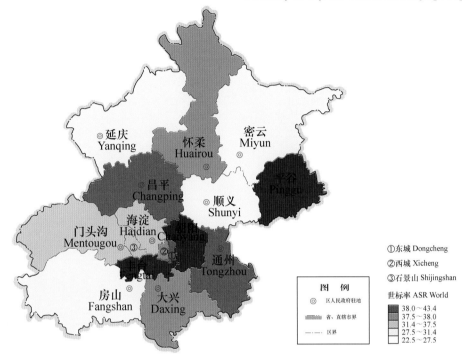

图 5.20.7 2019 年北京市户籍居民甲状腺癌世标发病率（1/10^5）地区分布情况
Figure 5.20.7 ASRs World for incidence of thyroid cancer（1/10^5）by district in Beijing, 2019

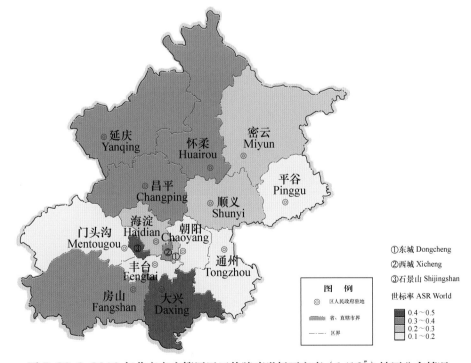

图 5.20.8 2019 年北京市户籍居民甲状腺癌世标死亡率（1/10^5）地区分布情况
Figure 5.20.8 ASRs World for mortality of thyroid cancer（1/10^5）by district in Beijing, 2019

（撰稿 杨雷，校稿 李晴雨）

5.21 淋巴瘤（C81-85, C88, C90, C96）

2019 年，北京市淋巴瘤新发病例数为 1 662 例，占全部恶性肿瘤发病的 2.85%，位居恶性肿瘤发病第 10 位；其中男性 919 例，女性 743 例，城区 1 121 例，郊区 541 例。淋巴瘤发病率为 11.99/10 万，中标发病率为 6.29/10 万，世标发病率为 6.06/10 万；男性世标发病率为女性的 1.26 倍，城区世标发病率为郊区的 1.20 倍。0~74 岁累积发病率为 0.67%（表 5.21.1）。

5.21 Lymphoma（C81-85, C88, C90, C96）

There were 1,662 new cases diagnosed as lymphoma（919 males and 743 females, 1,121 in urban areas and 541 in peri-urban areas）, accounting for 2.85% of new cases of all cancers in 2019. Lymphoma was the 10th common cancer in Beijing. The crude incidence rate was 11.99 per 100,000, with an ASR China and an ASR World of 6.29 and 6.06 per 100,000, respectively. The ASR World for incidence was 26% higher in males than in females and 20% higher in urban areas than in peri-urban areas. The cumulative incidence rate for subjects aged 0 to 74 years was 0.67%（Table 5.21.1）.

表 5.21.1 2019 年北京市户籍居民淋巴瘤发病情况
Table 5.21.1 Incidence of lymphoma in Beijing, 2019

地区 Area	性别 Sex	例数 No. of cases	粗率 Crude rate （1/10⁵）	构成比 Freq.（%）	中标率 ASR China （1/10⁵）	世标率 ASR World （1/10⁵）	累积率 Cumulative rate（0~74, %）	顺位 Rank
全市 All areas	合计 Both	1 662	11.99	2.85	6.29	6.06	0.67	10
	男性 Male	919	13.33	3.22	7.04	6.80	0.75	10
	女性 Female	743	10.66	2.50	5.61	5.38	0.59	10
城区 Urban areas	合计 Both	1 121	13.12	2.94	6.70	6.48	0.71	10
	男性 Male	616	14.52	3.33	7.48	7.20	0.77	9
	女性 Female	505	11.74	2.58	5.99	5.81	0.64	10
郊区 Peri-urban areas	合计 Both	541	10.16	2.68	5.62	5.38	0.60	10
	男性 Male	303	11.42	3.01	6.29	6.13	0.70	10
	女性 Female	238	8.91	2.36	5.02	4.71	0.50	10

2019 年，北京市淋巴瘤死亡病例数为 1 020 例，占全部恶性肿瘤死亡的 3.73%，位居恶性肿瘤死亡第 8 位；其中男性 589 例，女性 431 例，城区 704 例，郊区 316 例。淋巴瘤死亡率为 7.36/10 万，中标死亡率为 3.02/10 万，世标死亡率为 2.98/10 万；男性世标死亡率为女性的 1.49 倍，城区世标死亡率为郊区的 1.07 倍。0~74 岁累积死亡率为 0.33%（表 5.21.2）。

A total of 1,020 cases died of lymphoma（589 males and 431 females, 704 in urban areas and 316 in peri-urban areas）, accounting for 3.73% of all cancer deaths in 2019. Lymphoma was the 8th leading cause of cancer deaths in all cancers. The crude mortality rate was 7.36 per 100,000, with an ASR China and an ASR World of 3.02 and 2.98 per 100,000, respectively. The ASR World for mortality was 49% higher in males than in females and 7% higher in urban areas than in peri-urban areas. The cumulative mortality rate for subjects aged 0 to 74 years was 0.33%（Table 5.21.2）.

表 5.21.2 2019 年北京市户籍居民淋巴瘤死亡情况
Table 5.21.2 Mortality of lymphoma in Beijing, 2019

地区 Area	性别 Sex	例数 No. of deaths	粗率 Crude rate （1/10⁵）	构成比 Freq.（%）	中标率 ASR China （1/10⁵）	世标率 ASR World （1/10⁵）	累积率 Cumulative rate（0~74, %）	顺位 Rank
全市 All areas	合计 Both	1 020	7.36	3.73	3.02	2.98	0.33	8
	男性 Male	589	8.54	3.64	3.64	3.61	0.40	9
	女性 Female	431	6.18	3.87	2.45	2.41	0.27	9
城区 Urban areas	合计 Both	704	8.24	3.94	3.09	3.03	0.33	7
	男性 Male	402	9.48	3.88	3.56	3.52	0.38	9
	女性 Female	302	7.02	4.04	2.68	2.59	0.29	8
郊区 Peri-urban areas	合计 Both	316	5.94	3.33	2.83	2.84	0.33	8
	男性 Male	187	7.05	3.20	3.65	3.62	0.44	8
	女性 Female	129	4.83	3.52	2.06	2.11	0.23	9

北 京 市 淋 巴 瘤 世 标 发 病 率 2010 年 为 5.71/10 万，2019 年为 6.06/10 万，年均变化百分比为 -0.09%（P = 0.845）；男性和女性世标发

The ASR World for incidence of lymphoma was 5.71 per 100,000 in 2010 and 6.06 per 100,000 in 2019; and the APC of ASR World for incidence was -0.09%（P = 0.845）. The APCs of ASR World for incidence

病率 10 年间年均变化百分比分别为 0.31% （*P* = 0.502）和 - 0.53%（*P* = 0.439）。北京市淋巴瘤世标死亡率 2010 年为 2.90/10 万，2019 年为 2.98/10 万，年均变化百分比为 - 0.20% （*P* = 0.534）；男性和女性世标死亡率 10 年间年均变化百分比分别为 0.05%（*P* = 0.911）和 - 0.46%（*P* = 0.578）。

淋巴瘤年龄别发病率在 45 岁之前处于较低水平，45 岁以后快速上升；淋巴瘤年龄别死亡率在 50 岁之前处于较低水平，自 50 岁开始快速上升。淋巴瘤发病率和死亡率分别在 80～84 岁与 85 岁及以上年龄组达到高峰（图 5.21.1 至图 5.21.6）。50 岁及以上各年龄组男性发病率和死亡率均高于女性（图 5.21.1 和图 5.21.4）。城区和郊区年龄别发病率、死亡率变化总体趋势类似，但郊区死亡率波动更明显（图 5.21.2 和图 5.21.3，图 5.21.5 和图 5.21.6）。

of lymphoma in males and females were 0.31% （*P* = 0.502）and - 0.53%（*P* = 0.439）, respectively. The ASR World for mortality of lymphoma was 2.90 per 100,000 in 2010 and 2.98 per 100,000 in 2019; and the APC of ASR World for mortality was - 0.20% （*P* = 0.534）. The APCs of ASR World for mortality of lymphoma in males and females were 0.05% （*P* = 0.911）and - 0.46%（*P* = 0.578）, respectively.

The age-specific incidence rate of lymphoma was relatively low in people below 45 years old, and thereafter increased sharply with advancing age. The age-specific mortality rate of lymphoma was relatively low before 50 years old and gradually increased with advancing age. The age-specific incidence and mortality rates of lymphoma reached the peak at the age group of 80-84 years and 85 years and above, respectively（Figure 5.21.1-5.21.6）. The incidence and mortality rates in males were higher than those in females after 50 years old（Figure 5.21.1, Figure 5.21.4）. The overall trends of age-specific incidence and mortality rates in urban and peri-urban areas were same, but the mortality rates in peri-urban areas showed huge fluctuations（Figure 5.21.2-5.21.3, Figure 5.21.5-5.21.6）.

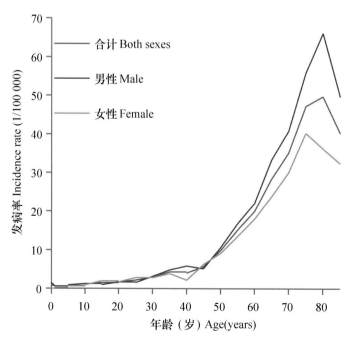

图 5.21.1 2019 年北京市户籍居民淋巴瘤年龄别发病率
Figure 5.21.1 Age-specific incidence rates of lymphoma in Beijing, 2019

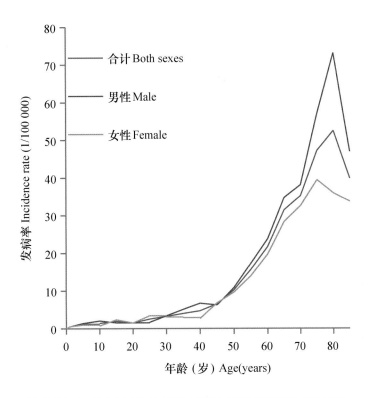

图 5.21.2 2019 年北京市城区户籍居民淋巴瘤年龄别发病率
Figure 5.21.2 Age-specific incidence rates of lymphoma in urban areas of Beijing, 2019

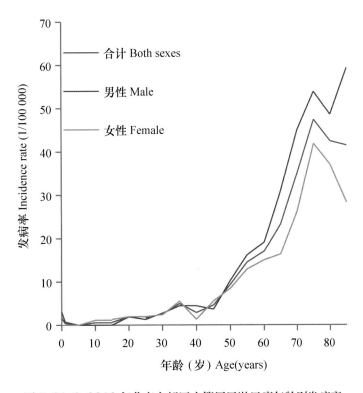

图 5.21.3 2019 年北京市郊区户籍居民淋巴瘤年龄别发病率
Figure 5.21.3 Age-specific incidence rates of lymphoma in peri-urban areas of Beijing, 2019

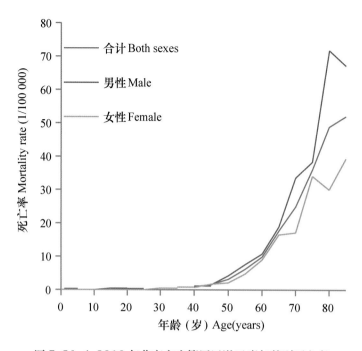

图 5.21.4 2019 年北京市户籍居民淋巴瘤年龄别死亡率
Figure 5.21.4 Age-specific mortality rates of lymphoma in Beijing, 2019

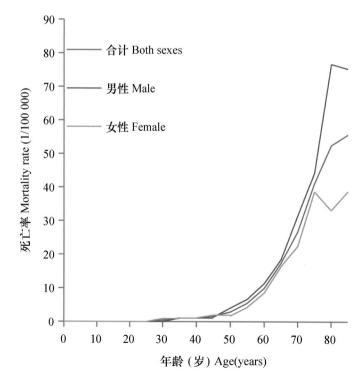

图 5.21.5 2019 年北京市城区户籍居民淋巴瘤年龄别死亡率
Figure 5.21.5 Age-specific mortality rates of lymphoma in urban areas of Beijing, 2019

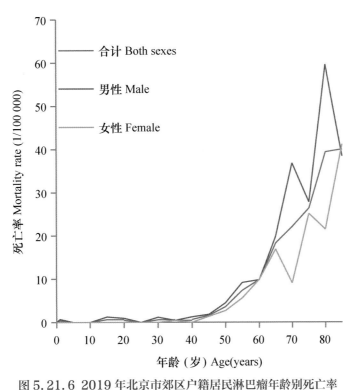

图 5.21.6 2019 年北京市郊区户籍居民淋巴瘤年龄别死亡率
Figure 5.21.6 Age-specific mortality rates of lymphoma in peri-urban areas of Beijing, 2019

2019 年，北京市淋巴瘤世标发病率在 16 个辖区间有差异，城区发病率高于郊区；世标死亡率在 16 个辖区间差异不明显（图 5.21.7 和图 5.21.8）。

In 2019, there were differences among the 16 districts in ASR World for incidence of lymphoma in Beijing. The incidence rate was higher in urban areas than in peri-urban areas. There was a slight difference among the 16 districts in ASR World for mortality of lymphoma in Beijing（Figure 5.21.7-5.21.8）.

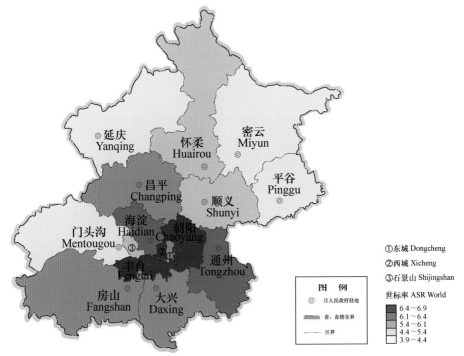

图 5.21.7 2019 年北京市户籍居民淋巴瘤世标发病率（1/10^5）地区分布情况
Figure 5.21.7 ASRs World for incidence of lymphoma（1/10^5）by district in Beijing, 2019

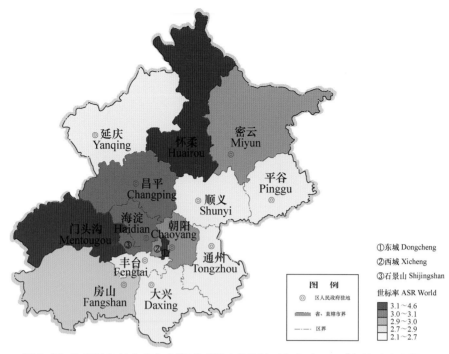

图 5.21.8 2019 年北京市户籍居民淋巴瘤世标死亡率（1/10⁵）地区分布情况
Figure 5.21.8 ASRs World for mortality of lymphoma（1/10⁵）by district in Beijing, 2019

全部淋巴瘤病例中有明确病理分型的占 98.37%。其中弥漫性非霍奇金淋巴瘤是最主要的病理类型，占 28.88%；其后依次是非霍奇金淋巴瘤的其他和未特指类型（25.45%）、多发性骨髓瘤和恶性浆细胞肿瘤（24.67%）、滤泡性非霍奇金淋巴瘤（8.72%）、周围和皮肤 T 细胞淋巴瘤（6.14%）、霍奇金淋巴瘤（3.85%）和恶性免疫增生性疾病（0.66%）（图 5.21.9）。

Among all lymphoma cases, 98.37% had morphological verification. Among them, the diffuse non-Hodgkin lymphoma was the most common histological type, accounting for 28.88% of all cases, followed by other and unspecified types of non-Hodgkin lymphoma（25.45%）, the multiple myeloma and malignant plasma cell neoplasms（24.67%）, the follicular non-Hodgkin lymphoma（8.72%）, the peripheral and cutaneous T-cell lymphoma（6.14%）, the Hodgkin lymphoma（3.85%）, and the malignant immunoproliferative disease（0.66%）（Figure 5.21.9）.

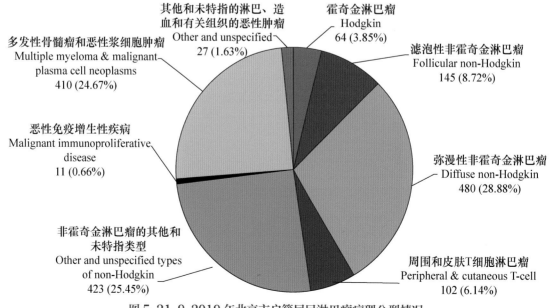

图 5.21.9 2019 年北京市户籍居民淋巴瘤病理分型情况
Figure 5.21.9 Morphological distribution of lymphoma in Beijing, 2019

（撰稿 李浩鑫，校稿 张希）

5.22 白血病（C91-95, D45-47）

2019 年，北京市白血病新发病例数为 1 286 例，占全部恶性肿瘤发病的 2.21%，位居恶性肿瘤发病第 13 位；其中男性 743 例，女性 543 例，城区 802 例，郊区 484 例。白血病发病率为 9.27/10 万，中标发病率为 5.53/10 万，世标发病率为 5.82/10 万；男性世标发病率为女性的 1.34 倍，郊区世标发病率为城区的 1.18 倍。0~74 岁累积发病率为 0.53%（表 5.22.1）。

5.22 Leukemia（C91-95, D45-47）

There were 1,286 new cases diagnosed as leukemia (743 males and 543 females, 802 in urban areas and 484 in peri-urban areas), accounting for 2.21% of new cases of all cancers in 2019. Leukemia was the 13th common cancer in Beijing. The crude incidence rate was 9.27 per 100,000, with an ASR China and an ASR World of 5.53 and 5.82 per 100,000, respectively. The ASR World for incidence was 34% higher in males than in females and 18% higher in peri-urban areas than in urban areas. The cumulative incidence rate for subjects aged 0 to 74 years was 0.53%（Table 5.22.1）.

表 5.22.1 2019 年北京市户籍居民白血病发病情况
Table 5.22.1 Incidence of leukemia in Beijing, 2019

地区 Area	性别 Sex	例数 No. of cases	粗率 Crude rate （1/10^5）	构成比 Freq.（%）	中标率 ASR China （1/10^5）	世标率 ASR World （1/10^5）	累积率 Cumulative rate（0~74, %）	顺位 Rank
全市 All areas	合计 Both	1 286	9.27	2.21	5.53	5.82	0.53	13
	男性 Male	743	10.78	2.60	6.41	6.70	0.63	12
	女性 Female	543	7.79	1.83	4.72	5.01	0.45	14
城区 Urban areas	合计 Both	802	9.39	2.11	5.19	5.44	0.50	13
	男性 Male	475	11.20	2.57	6.10	6.36	0.60	12
	女性 Female	327	7.60	1.67	4.37	4.60	0.40	14
郊区 Peri-urban areas	合计 Both	484	9.09	2.40	6.06	6.41	0.59	13
	男性 Male	268	10.10	2.66	6.87	7.22	0.67	12
	女性 Female	216	8.09	2.14	5.29	5.64	0.52	13

2019 年，北京市白血病死亡病例数为 957 例，占全部恶性肿瘤死亡的 3.50%，位居恶性肿瘤死亡第 10 位；其中男性 599 例，女性 358 例，城区 646 例，郊区 311 例。白血病死亡率为 6.90/10 万，中标发病率为 3.23/10 万，世标发病率为 3.16/10 万；男性世标死亡率为女性的 1.80 倍，郊区世标死亡率为城区的 1.01 倍。0~74 岁累积死亡率为 0.32%（表 5.22.2）。

A total of 957 cases died of leukemia（599 males and 358 females, 646 in urban areas and 311 in peri-urban areas）, accounting for 3.50% of all cancer deaths in 2019. Leukemia was the 10th leading cause of cancer deaths in all cancers. The crude mortality rate was 6.90 per 100,000, with an ASR China and an ASR World of 3.23 and 3.16 per 100,000, respectively. The ASR World for mortality was 80% higher in males than in females and 1% higher in peri-urban areas than in urban areas. The cumulative mortality rate for subjects aged 0 to 74 years was 0.32%（Table 5.22.2）.

表 5.22.2　2019 年北京市户籍居民白血病死亡情况
Table 5.22.2 Mortality of leukemia in Beijing, 2019

地区 Area	性别 Sex	例数 No. of deaths	粗率 Crude rate （1/10^5）	构成比 Freq.（%）	中标率 ASR China （1/10^5）	世标率 ASR World （1/10^5）	累积率 Cumulative rate（0~74, %）	顺位 Rank
全市 All areas	合计 Both	957	6.90	3.50	3.23	3.16	0.32	10
	男性 Male	599	8.69	3.70	4.17	4.11	0.43	8
	女性 Female	358	5.14	3.21	2.36	2.28	0.23	10
城区 Urban areas	合计 Both	646	7.56	3.62	3.16	3.13	0.32	8
	男性 Male	417	9.83	4.02	4.28	4.27	0.43	8
	女性 Female	229	5.32	3.06	2.14	2.08	0.22	11
郊区 Peri-urban areas	合计 Both	311	5.84	3.27	3.26	3.15	0.33	9
	男性 Male	182	6.86	3.12	3.89	3.80	0.42	10
	女性 Female	129	4.83	3.52	2.68	2.57	0.25	10

北京市白血病世标发病率 2010 年为 5.17/10 万，2019 年[1]为 5.82/10 万，年均变化百分比为 0.97%（P=0.424）；男性和女性世标发病率

The ASR World for incidence of leukemia was 5.17 per 100,000 in 2010, and 5.82 per 100,000 in 2019[2]; the APC of ASR World for incidence was 0.97%（P= 0.424）. The APCs of ASR World for incidence of

① 2010—2016 年白血病统计范围为 ICD-10 编码 C91-95，2017—2019 年统计范围为 C91-95 和 D45-47。

② Codes C91-95 in the ICD-10 were included in the analysis as leukemia from 2010 to 2016. Codes C91-95 and D45-47 were included in the analysis as leukemia in 2017-2019.

10 年间年均变化百分比分别为 1.12%（P = 0.334）和 0.89%（P = 0.546）。北京市白血病世标死亡率 2010 年为 3.33/10 万，2019 年为 3.16/10 万，年均变化百分比为 −0.42%（P = 0.712）；男性和女性世标死亡率 10 年间年均变化百分比分别为 0.62%（P = 0.626）和 −1.86%（P = 0.150）。

白血病年龄别发病率在 0～4 岁组较高，在 5 岁后趋于平缓，从 50～54 岁组开始快速升高，在 80～84 岁组达到高峰（图 5.22.1 至图 5.22.3）。白血病年龄别死亡率在 50 岁之前均处于较低水平，自 50 岁后开始快速升高，在 85 岁及以上年龄组达到高峰（图 5.22.4 至图 5.22.6）。60 岁后，男性发病率和死亡率均显著高于女性（图 5.22.1 和图 5.22.4）。城区和郊区年龄别发病率和死亡率变化有一定差异，但总体趋势相同（图 5.22.2 和图 5.22.3，图 5.22.5 和图 5.22.6）。

leukemia in males and females were 1.12%（P = 0.334）and 0.89%（P = 0.546）, respectively. The ASR World for mortality of leukemia was 3.33 per 100,000 in 2010 and 3.16 per 100,000 in 2019; the APC of ASR World for mortality was −0.42%（P = 0.712）. The APCs of ASR World for mortality of leukemia in males and females were 0.62%（P = 0.626）and −1.86%（P = 0.150）, respectively.

The age-specific incidence rate was relatively high at the age group of 0-4 years, and remained relatively stable since 5 years old. It dramatically increased at the age group of 50-54 years, and peaked at the age group of 80-84 years（Figure 5.22.1-5.22.3）. The age-specific mortality rate was at low level in age below 50 years, and thereafter increased rapidly, peaking at the age group of 85 years and above（Figure 5.22.4-5.22.6）. The incidence and mortality rates in males were significantly higher than those in females after 60 years old（Figure 5.22.1, Figure 5.22.4）. There were some differences in age-specific incidence and mortality rates between urban and peri-urban areas, but the overall trends were same（Figure 5.22.2-5.22.3, Figure 5.22.5-5.22.6）.

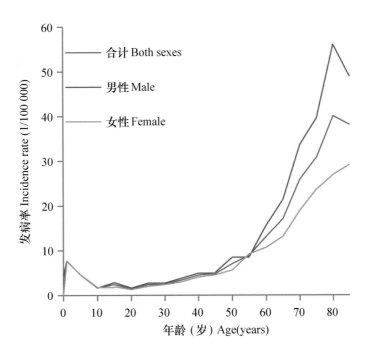

图 5.22.1 2019 年北京市户籍居民白血病年龄别发病率
Figure 5.22.1 Age-specific incidence rates of leukemia in Beijing, 2019

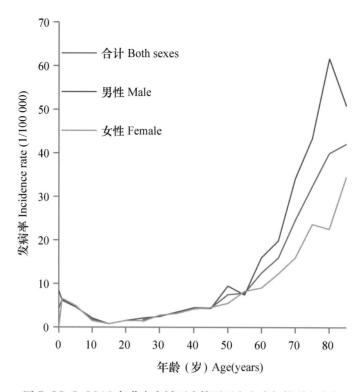

图 5.22.2 2019 年北京市城区户籍居民白血病年龄别发病率
Figure 5.22.2 Age-specific incidence rates of leukemia in urban areas of Beijing, 2019

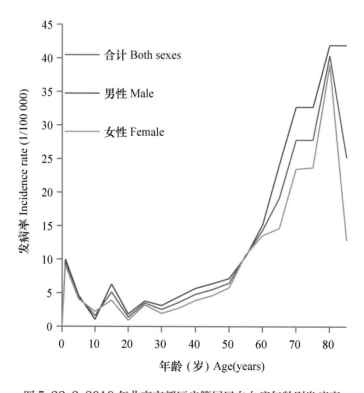

图 5.22.3 2019 年北京市郊区户籍居民白血病年龄别发病率
Figure 5.22.3 Age-specific incidence rates of leukemia in peri-urban areas of Beijing, 2019

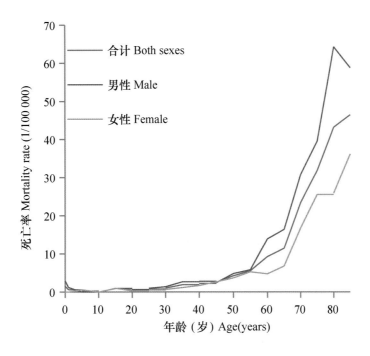

图 5.22.4 2019 年北京市户籍居民白血病年龄别死亡率
Figure 5.22.4 Age-specific mortality rates of leukemia in Beijing, 2019

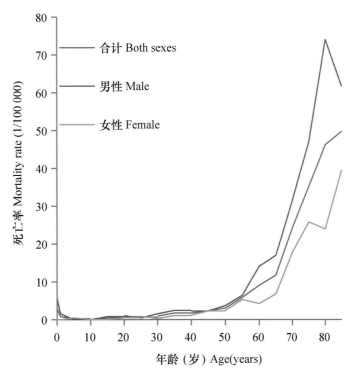

图 5.22.5 2019 年北京市城区户籍居民白血病年龄别死亡率
Figure 5.22.5 Age-specific mortality rates of leukemia in urban areas of Beijing, 2019

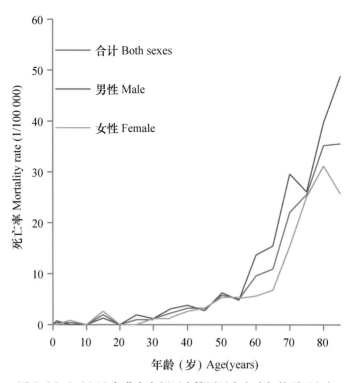

图 5.22.6 2019 年北京市郊区户籍居民白血病年龄别死亡率
Figure 5.22.6 Age-specific mortality rates of leukemia in peri-urban areas of Beijing, 2019

白血病（C91-95）新发病例（926 例）中，最主要的病理类型是髓样白血病，占 52.70%；其后依次为淋巴样白血病（25.16%）和未特指细胞类型的白血病（15.44%）（图 5.22.7）。

Among the 926 new cases of leukemia（C91-95）, myeloid leukemia was the most common histological type, accounting for 52.70%, followed by lymphoid leukemia（25.16%）and unspecified cell type leukemia（15.44%）（Figure 5.22.7）.

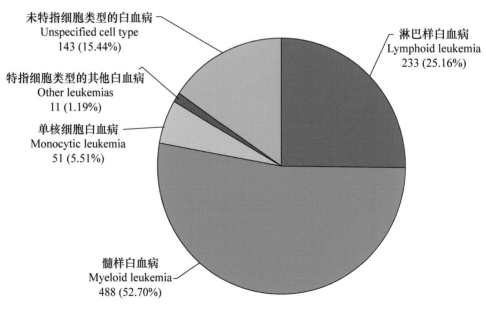

图 5.22.7 2019 年北京市户籍居民白血病（C91-95）病理分型情况
Figure 5.22.7 Morphological distribution of leukemia （C91-95） in Beijing, 2019

（撰稿 李浩鑫，校稿 张希）

5.23 皮肤恶性黑色素瘤（C43）[1]

2019 年，北京市皮肤恶性黑色素瘤新发病例数为 130 例，占全部恶性肿瘤发病的 0.22%，位居恶性肿瘤发病第 23 位；其中男性 57 例，女性 73 例，城区 84 例，郊区 46 例。皮肤恶性黑色素瘤发病率为 0.94/10 万，中标发病率为 0.51/10 万，世标发病率为 0.48/10 万；女性世标发病率为男性的 1.33 倍，城区世标发病率为郊区的 1.06 倍。0~74 岁累积发病率为 0.05%（表 5.23.1）。

5.23 Cutaneous malignant melanoma（C43）[2]

There were 130 new cases diagnosed as cutaneous malignant melanoma（57 males and 73 females, 84 in urban areas and 46 in peri-urban areas）, accounting for 0.22% of new cases of all cancers in 2019. Cutaneous malignant melanoma was the 23rd common cancer in Beijing. The crude incidence rate was 0.94 per 100,000, with an ASR China and an ASR World of 0.51 and 0.48 per 100,000, respectively. The ASR World for incidence was 33% higher in females than in males and 6% higher in urban areas than in peri-urban areas. The cumulative incidence rate for subjects aged 0 to 74 years was 0.05%（Table 5.23.1）.

表 5.23.1 2019 年北京市户籍居民皮肤恶性黑色素瘤发病情况
Table 5.23.1 Incidence of cutaneous malignant melanoma in Beijing, 2019

地区 Area	性别 Sex	例数 No. of cases	粗率 Crude rate （1/10^5）	构成比 Freq.（%）	中标率 ASR China （1/10^5）	世标率 ASR World （1/10^5）	累积率 Cumulative rate（0~74, %）	顺位 Rank
全市 All areas	合计 Both	130	0.94	0.22	0.51	0.48	0.05	23
	男性 Male	57	0.83	0.20	0.41	0.41	0.04	20
	女性 Female	73	1.05	0.25	0.59	0.54	0.06	19
城区 Urban areas	合计 Both	84	0.98	0.22	0.52	0.49	0.05	23
	男性 Male	34	0.80	0.18	0.37	0.36	0.04	20
	女性 Female	50	1.16	0.26	0.67	0.62	0.06	19
郊区 Peri-urban areas	合计 Both	46	0.86	0.23	0.48	0.46	0.05	23
	男性 Male	23	0.87	0.23	0.48	0.49	0.05	19
	女性 Female	23	0.86	0.23	0.48	0.43	0.05	20

---

[1] 因北京市皮肤恶性黑色素瘤发病和死亡例数较少，本节不包含年龄别发病率和死亡率的统计数据及图表。

[2] Because of few cutaneous malignant melanoma cases and deaths occurred in Beijing in 2019, this section does not contain statistical data and charts on age-specific incidence and mortality rates.

2019 年，北京市皮肤恶性黑色素瘤死亡病例数为 71 例，占全部恶性肿瘤死亡的 0.26%，位居恶性肿瘤死亡第 24 位；其中男性 36 例，女性 35 例，城区 52 例，郊区 19 例。皮肤恶性黑色素瘤死亡率为 0.51/10 万，中标死亡率为 0.23/10 万，世标死亡率为 0.22/10 万；女性世标死亡率为男性的 1.11 倍，城区世标死亡率是郊区的 1.53 倍。0～74 岁累积死亡率为 0.02%（表 5.23.2）。

A total of 71 cases died of cutaneous malignant melanoma（36 males and 35 females, 52 in urban areas and 19 in peri-urban areas）, accounting for 0.26% of all cancer deaths in 2019. Cutaneous malignant melanoma was the 24th leading cause of cancer deaths in all cancers. The crude mortality rate was 0.51 per 100,000, with an ASR China and an ASR World of 0.23 and 0.22 per 100,000, respectively. The ASR World for mortality was 11% higher in females than in males and 53% higher in urban areas than in peri-urban areas. The cumulative mortality rate for subjects aged 0 to 74 years was 0.02%（Table 5.23.2）.

表 5.23.2 2019 年北京市户籍居民皮肤恶性黑色素瘤死亡情况
Table 5.23.2 Mortality of cutaneous malignant melanoma in Beijing, 2019

地区 Area	性别 Sex	例数 No. of deaths	粗率 Crude rate （1/10^5）	构成比 Freq.（%）	中标率 ASR China （1/10^5）	世标率 ASR World （1/10^5）	累积率 Cumulative rate（0~74, %）	顺位 Rank
全市 All areas	合计 Both	71	0.51	0.26	0.23	0.22	0.02	24
	男性 Male	36	0.52	0.22	0.21	0.21	0.03	19
	女性 Female	35	0.50	0.31	0.26	0.24	0.02	20
城区 Urban areas	合计 Both	52	0.61	0.29	0.28	0.26	0.03	24
	男性 Male	26	0.61	0.25	0.24	0.24	0.03	19
	女性 Female	26	0.60	0.35	0.32	0.28	0.03	20
郊区 Peri-urban areas	合计 Both	19	0.36	0.20	0.16	0.17	0.02	24
	男性 Male	10	0.38	0.17	0.16	0.18	0.02	20
	女性 Female	9	0.34	0.25	0.17	0.16	0.01	20

北京市皮肤恶性黑色素瘤世标发病率 2010 年为 0.42/10 万，2019 年为 0.48/10 万，年均变化百分比为 - 1.39%（$P=0.541$）；男性和女性世标发病率 10 年间年均变化百分比分别为 - 2.36%（$P=0.496$）和 - 0.52%（$P=0.769$）。北京市皮肤恶性黑色素瘤世标死亡率 2010 年为 0.17/10 万，2019 年为 0.22/10 万，年均变化百分比为 0.83%（$P=0.527$）；男性和女性世标死亡率 10 年间年均变化百分比分别为 - 0.50%（$P=0.797$）和 2.71%（$P=0.257$）。

The ASR World for incidence of cutaneous malignant melanoma was 0.42 per 100,000 in 2010 and 0.48 per 100,000 in 2019; and the APC of ASR World for incidence was - 1.39%（$P=0.541$）. The APCs of ASR World for incidence of cutaneous malignant melanoma in males and females were - 2.36%（$P=0.496$）and - 0.52%（$P=0.769$）, respectively. The ASR World for mortality of cutaneous malignant melanoma was 0.17 per 100,000 in 2010 and 0.22 per 100,000 in 2019; and the APC of ASR World for mortality was 0.83%（$P=0.572$）. The APCs of ASR World for mortality of cutaneous malignant melanoma in males and females were - 0.50%（$P=0.797$）and 2.71%（$P=0.257$）, respectively.

（撰稿 刘硕，校稿 李慧超）

附　录
Appendix

附表 1　2019 年北京市户籍居民恶性肿瘤发病主要指标
Appendix table 1 Incidence of all cancers in Beijing, 2019

部位 Site	男性 Male					
	例数 No. of cases	粗率 Crude rate （1/10^5）	构成比 Freq. （%）	中标率 ASR China （1/10^5）	世标率 ASR World （1/10^5）	累积率 Cumulative rate （0~74，%）
口腔和咽 Oral cavity & pharynx	493	7.15	1.73	3.58	3.57	0.43
鼻咽 Nasopharynx	64	0.93	0.22	0.61	0.58	0.06
食管 Esophagus	933	13.53	3.27	5.97	6.11	0.73
胃 Stomach	1 820	26.40	6.37	11.82	11.75	1.39
结直肠 Colon-rectum	4 348	63.06	15.22	29.35	29.25	3.57
肝 Liver	1750	25.38	6.13	12.38	12.41	1.43
胆囊 Gallbladder	651	9.44	2.28	4.05	4.07	0.46
胰腺 Pancreas	802	11.63	2.81	5.24	5.26	0.63
喉 Larynx	302	4.38	1.06	2.04	2.10	0.26
肺 Lung	7 148	103.68	25.02	47.00	47.01	5.86
其他胸腔器官 Other thoracic organs	103	1.49	0.36	0.92	0.94	0.10
骨 Bone	88	1.28	0.31	0.84	0.82	0.07
皮肤恶性黑色素瘤 Cutaneous malignant melanoma	57	0.83	0.20	0.41	0.41	0.04
乳腺 Breast	34	0.49	0.12	0.24	0.24	0.03
子宫颈 Cervix	—	—	—	—	—	—
子宫体 Uterus	—	—	—	—	—	—
卵巢 Ovary	—	—	—	—	—	—
前列腺 Prostate	1 798	26.08	6.29	11.04	10.86	1.33
睾丸 Testis	47	0.68	0.16	0.70	0.67	0.05
肾及泌尿系统部位不明 Kidney & unspecified urinary organs	1 504	21.81	5.26	11.71	11.55	1.36
膀胱 Bladder	1 473	21.36	5.16	9.45	9.42	1.16
脑 Brain	438	6.35	1.53	4.50	4.41	0.41
甲状腺 Thyroid	1 799	26.09	6.30	25.10	20.30	1.75
淋巴瘤 Lymphoma	919	13.33	3.22	7.04	6.80	0.75
白血病 Leukemia	743	10.78	2.60	6.41	6.70	0.63
其他 Other	1 257	18.23	4.40	9.10	9.29	0.97
所有部位合计 All sites	28 571	414.40	100.00	209.50	204.52	23.47
所有部位除外皮肤 All sites exc. C44	28 266	409.97	98.93	207.40	202.45	23.26

	女性 Female					
例数 No. of cases	粗率 Crude rate （1/10⁵）	构成比 Freq. （%）	中标率 ASR China （1/10⁵）	世标率 ASR World （1/10⁵）	累积率 Cumulative rate （0~74，%）	ICD10
276	3.96	0.93	2.12	1.99	0.20	C00-10, C12-14
29	0.42	0.10	0.23	0.21	0.02	C11
257	3.69	0.87	1.18	1.21	0.12	C15
815	11.69	2.75	5.21	5.00	0.54	C16
3 001	43.05	10.12	19.02	18.56	2.17	C18-21
635	9.11	2.14	3.53	3.60	0.38	C22
589	8.45	1.99	3.19	3.14	0.35	C23-24
773	11.09	2.61	4.28	4.24	0.46	C25
17	0.24	0.06	0.10	0.10	0.01	C32
5 498	78.86	18.53	36.38	35.64	4.13	C33-34
57	0.82	0.19	0.48	0.50	0.05	C37-38
65	0.93	0.22	0.62	0.60	0.06	C40-41
73	1.05	0.25	0.59	0.54	0.06	C43
5 949	85.33	20.06	52.17	48.92	5.37	C50
659	9.45	2.22	6.65	5.94	0.61	C53
1 523	21.85	5.13	12.79	12.38	1.43	C54-55
851	12.21	2.87	7.59	7.26	0.79	C56
—	—	—	—	—	—	C61
—	—	—	—	—	—	C62
875	12.55	2.95	5.91	5.72	0.64	C64-66, C68
449	6.44	1.51	2.57	2.51	0.30	C67
356	5.11	1.20	3.68	3.70	0.31	C70-C72
4 445	63.76	14.98	58.73	49.27	4.36	C73
743	10.66	2.50	5.61	5.38	0.59	C81-85, C88, C90, C96
543	7.79	1.83	4.72	5.01	0.45	C91-95, D45-47
1185	17.00	3.99	8.13	8.26	0.86	Other
29 663	425.48	100.00	245.48	229.68	24.25	All
29 344	420.90	98.92	243.53	227.74	24.03	All sites exc. C44

附表 2　2019 年北京市户籍居民恶性肿瘤死亡主要指标
Appendix table 2　Mortality of all cancers in Beijing, 2019

部位 Site	男性 Male					
	例数 No. of deaths	粗率 Crude rate （1/10⁵）	构成比 Freq. （%）	中标率 ASR China （1/10⁵）	世标率 ASR World （1/10⁵）	累积率 Cumulative rate （0~74，%）
口腔和咽 Oral cavity & pharynx	265	3.84	1.64	1.69	1.74	0.21
鼻咽 Nasopharynx	66	0.96	0.41	0.51	0.49	0.05
食管 Esophagus	805	11.68	4.97	4.91	5.02	0.58
胃 Stomach	1 307	18.96	8.07	7.64	7.64	0.84
结直肠 Colon-rectum	1 812	26.28	11.18	10.50	10.41	1.02
肝 Liver	1 424	20.65	8.79	9.62	9.60	1.10
胆囊 Gallbladder	535	7.76	3.30	3.16	3.17	0.35
胰腺 Pancreas	739	10.72	4.56	4.67	4.69	0.55
喉 Larynx	138	2.00	0.85	0.78	0.80	0.09
肺 Lung	5 112	74.15	31.55	30.78	30.64	3.48
其他胸腔器官 Other thoracic organs	71	1.03	0.44	0.59	0.58	0.06
骨 Bone	60	0.87	0.37	0.49	0.45	0.04
皮肤恶性黑色素瘤 Cutaneous malignant melanoma	36	0.52	0.22	0.21	0.21	0.03
乳腺 Breast	11	0.16	0.07	0.07	0.06	0.00
子宫颈 Cervix	—	—	—	—	—	—
子宫体 Uterus	—	—	—	—	—	—
卵巢 Ovary	—	—	—	—	—	—
前列腺 Prostate	694	10.07	4.28	3.12	3.20	0.20
睾丸 Testis	7	0.10	0.04	0.08	0.08	0.00
肾及泌尿系统部位不明 Kidney & unspecified urinary organs	464	6.73	2.86	2.73	2.78	0.29
膀胱 Bladder	570	8.27	3.52	2.73	2.81	0.23
脑 Brain	293	4.25	1.81	2.36	2.38	0.25
甲状腺 Thyroid	32	0.46	0.20	0.22	0.21	0.03
淋巴瘤 Lymphoma	589	8.54	3.64	3.64	3.61	0.40
白血病 Leukemia	599	8.69	3.70	4.17	4.11	0.43
其他 Other	574	8.33	3.54	3.59	3.65	0.35
所有部位合计 All sites	16 203	235.01	100.00	98.25	98.31	10.57
所有部位除外皮肤 All sites exc. C44	16 125	233.88	99.52	97.89	97.92	10.55

			女性 Female			
例数 No. of deaths	粗率 Crude rate (1/10⁵)	构成比 Freq. (%)	中标率 ASR China (1/10⁵)	世标率 ASR World (1/10⁵)	累积率 Cumulative rate (0~74, %)	ICD10
98	1.41	0.88	0.53	0.50	0.05	C00-10, C12-14
22	0.32	0.20	0.15	0.14	0.02	C11
203	2.91	1.82	0.84	0.87	0.06	C15
600	8.61	5.38	3.39	3.26	0.31	C16
1 350	19.36	12.11	6.61	6.56	0.56	C18-21
542	7.77	4.86	2.75	2.75	0.29	C22
499	7.16	4.48	2.49	2.46	0.27	C23-24
706	10.13	6.33	3.65	3.61	0.37	C25
6	0.09	0.05	0.02	0.02	0.00	C32
2 698	38.70	24.20	13.35	13.09	1.23	C33-34
37	0.53	0.33	0.21	0.21	0.02	C37-38
34	0.49	0.31	0.29	0.28	0.02	C40-41
35	0.50	0.31	0.26	0.24	0.02	C43
1 167	16.74	10.47	7.38	7.23	0.77	C50
244	3.50	2.19	1.91	1.81	0.18	C53
239	3.43	2.14	1.53	1.51	0.19	C54-55
486	6.97	4.36	3.28	3.27	0.39	C56
—	—	—	—	—	—	C61
—	—	—	—	—	—	C62
311	4.46	2.79	1.41	1.41	0.12	C64-66, C68
187	2.68	1.68	0.83	0.84	0.08	C67
278	3.99	2.49	2.07	2.03	0.21	C70-C72
75	1.08	0.67	0.41	0.39	0.04	C73
431	6.18	3.87	2.45	2.41	0.27	C81-85, C88, C90, C96
358	5.14	3.21	2.36	2.28	0.23	C91-95, D45-47
541	7.76	4.85	3.06	3.05	0.30	Other
11 147	159.89	100.00	61.23	60.23	5.98	All
11 096	159.16	99.54	61.04	60.02	5.97	All sites exc. C44

附表 3 2019 年北京市城区户籍居民恶性肿瘤发病主要指标

Appendix table 3 Incidence of all cancers in urban areas of Beijing, 2019

部位 Site	男性 Male					
	例数 No. of cases	粗率 Crude rate （1/10⁵）	构成比 Freq. （%）	中标率 ASR China （1/10⁵）	世标率 ASR World （1/10⁵）	累积率 Cumulative rate （0~74，%）
口腔和咽 Oral cavity & pharynx	330	7.78	1.78	3.76	3.76	0.45
鼻咽 Nasopharynx	45	1.06	0.24	0.69	0.64	0.07
食管 Esophagus	513	12.09	2.77	4.94	5.15	0.60
胃 Stomach	1 220	28.76	6.60	12.08	12.03	1.45
结直肠 Colon-rectum	2 939	69.29	15.89	30.72	30.56	3.77
肝 Liver	1 042	24.56	5.63	11.18	11.26	1.31
胆囊 Gallbladder	361	8.51	1.95	3.36	3.34	0.36
胰腺 Pancreas	545	12.85	2.95	5.48	5.51	0.67
喉 Larynx	176	4.15	0.95	1.84	1.89	0.24
肺 Lung	4 403	103.80	23.80	45.01	45.03	5.64
其他胸腔器官 Other thoracic organs	72	1.70	0.39	1.05	1.04	0.10
骨 Bone	44	1.04	0.24	0.55	0.61	0.05
皮肤恶性黑色素瘤 Cutaneous malignant melanoma	34	0.80	0.18	0.37	0.36	0.04
乳腺 Breast	24	0.57	0.13	0.28	0.28	0.04
子宫颈 Cervix	—	—	—	—	—	—
子宫体 Uterus	—	—	—	—	—	—
卵巢 Ovary	—	—	—	—	—	—
前列腺 Prostate	1 337	31.52	7.23	12.65	12.45	1.55
睾丸 Testis	32	0.75	0.17	0.81	0.74	0.05
肾及泌尿系统部位不明 Kidney & unspecified urinary organs	1 017	23.98	5.50	12.43	12.11	1.45
膀胱 Bladder	970	22.87	5.24	9.49	9.45	1.15
脑 Brain	281	6.62	1.52	4.69	4.54	0.42
甲状腺 Thyroid	1 191	28.08	6.44	27.49	22.15	1.91
淋巴瘤 Lymphoma	616	14.52	3.33	7.48	7.20	0.77
白血病 Leukemia	475	11.20	2.57	6.10	6.36	0.60
其他 Other	831	19.59	4.49	9.08	9.44	0.96
所有部位合计 All sites	18 498	436.08	100.00	211.52	205.89	23.67
所有部位除外皮肤 All sites exc. C44	18 304	431.51	98.95	209.55	203.93	23.46

			女性 Female			
例数 No. of deaths	粗率 Crude rate (1/10⁵)	构成比 Freq. (%)	中标率 ASR China (1/10⁵)	世标率 ASR World (1/10⁵)	累积率 Cumulative rate (0~74, %)	ICD10
201	4.67	1.03	2.37	2.24	0.23	C00-10, C12-14
20	0.46	0.10	0.26	0.24	0.03	C11
140	3.25	0.72	0.94	0.96	0.10	C15
588	13.67	3.00	5.85	5.60	0.60	C16
2 026	47.10	10.35	19.56	19.14	2.25	C18-21
378	8.79	1.93	3.07	3.14	0.31	C22
376	8.74	1.92	3.10	3.06	0.36	C23-24
548	12.74	2.80	4.58	4.52	0.50	C25
10	0.23	0.05	0.10	0.09	0.01	C32
3 579	83.21	18.29	37.79	36.90	4.27	C33-34
37	0.86	0.19	0.53	0.57	0.06	C37-38
40	0.93	0.20	0.68	0.64	0.06	C40-41
50	1.16	0.26	0.67	0.62	0.06	C43
4 098	95.27	20.94	56.32	53.18	5.91	C50
402	9.35	2.05	6.54	5.92	0.61	C53
977	22.71	4.99	13.14	12.73	1.49	C54-55
559	13.00	2.86	8.16	7.79	0.83	C56
—	—	—	—	—	—	C61
—	—	—	—	—	—	C62
611	14.20	3.12	6.37	6.16	0.68	C64-66, C68
321	7.46	1.64	2.80	2.74	0.33	C67
241	5.60	1.23	4.16	4.25	0.35	C70-C72
2 756	64.07	14.08	60.09	50.19	4.47	C73
505	11.74	2.58	5.99	5.81	0.64	C81-85, C88, C90, C96
327	7.60	1.67	4.37	4.60	0.40	C91-95, D45-47
781	18.16	3.99	8.24	8.53	0.89	Other
19 571	455.00	100.00	255.66	239.63	25.42	All
19 361	450.11	98.93	253.65	237.60	25.20	All sites exc. C44

附表4 2019年北京市城区户籍居民恶性肿瘤死亡主要指标

Appendix table 4 Mortality of all cancers in urban areas of Beijing, 2019

部位 Site	男性 Male					
	例数 No. of deaths	粗率 Crude rate （1/10⁵）	构成比 Freq. （%）	中标率 ASR China （1/10⁵）	世标率 ASR World （1/10⁵）	累积率 Cumulative rate （0~74，%）
口腔和咽 Oral cavity & pharynx	169	3.98	1.63	1.68	1.71	0.20
鼻咽 Nasopharynx	42	0.99	0.41	0.46	0.46	0.05
食管 Esophagus	439	10.35	4.23	3.94	4.10	0.46
胃 Stomach	874	20.60	8.43	7.49	7.52	0.82
结直肠 Colon-rectum	1 243	29.30	11.99	10.71	10.67	1.11
肝 Liver	840	19.80	8.10	8.49	8.51	0.97
胆囊 Gallbladder	314	7.40	3.03	2.72	2.71	0.28
胰腺 Pancreas	502	11.83	4.84	4.83	4.89	0.58
喉 Larynx	80	1.89	0.77	0.67	0.70	0.08
肺 Lung	3 088	72.80	29.79	27.86	27.79	3.12
其他胸腔器官 Other thoracic organs	48	1.13	0.46	0.60	0.58	0.06
骨 Bone	34	0.80	0.33	0.45	0.42	0.03
皮肤恶性黑色素瘤 Cutaneous malignant melanoma	26	0.61	0.25	0.24	0.24	0.03
乳腺 Breast	7	0.17	0.07	0.06	0.05	0.00
子宫颈 Cervix	—	—	—	—	—	—
子宫体 Uterus	—	—	—	—	—	—
卵巢 Ovary	—	—	—	—	—	—
前列腺 Prostate	517	12.19	4.99	3.25	3.31	0.20
睾丸 Testis	6	0.14	0.06	0.09	0.09	0.00
肾及泌尿系统部位不明 Kidney & unspecified urinary organs	341	8.04	3.29	3.02	3.05	0.33
膀胱 Bladder	385	9.08	3.71	2.63	2.72	0.22
脑 Brain	185	4.36	1.78	2.18	2.31	0.24
甲状腺 Thyroid	16	0.38	0.15	0.16	0.16	0.02
淋巴瘤 Lymphoma	402	9.48	3.88	3.56	3.52	0.38
白血病 Leukemia	417	9.83	4.02	4.28	4.27	0.43
其他 Other	392	9.24	3.78	3.67	3.69	0.36
所有部位合计 All sites	10 367	244.40	100.00	93.03	93.43	9.97
所有部位除外皮肤 All sites exc. C44	10 313	243.12	99.48	92.69	93.07	9.95

例数 No. of deaths	粗率 Crude rate (1/10⁵)	构成比 Freq. (%)	中标率 ASR China (1/10⁵)	世标率 ASR World (1/10⁵)	累积率 Cumulative rate (0~74, %)	ICD10
		女性 Female				
70	1.63	0.94	0.56	0.54	0.05	C00-10, C12-14
16	0.37	0.21	0.20	0.18	0.02	C11
117	2.72	1.56	0.67	0.70	0.04	C15
421	9.79	5.63	3.51	3.39	0.32	C16
975	22.67	13.03	6.95	6.91	0.60	C18-21
325	7.56	4.34	2.38	2.40	0.22	C22
301	7.00	4.02	2.18	2.15	0.24	C23-24
512	11.90	6.84	3.95	3.91	0.40	C25
3	0.07	0.04	0.02	0.02	0.00	C32
1 677	38.99	22.42	11.79	11.54	1.03	C33-34
29	0.67	0.39	0.26	0.26	0.03	C37-38
22	0.51	0.29	0.27	0.25	0.02	C40-41
26	0.60	0.35	0.32	0.28	0.03	C43
864	20.09	11.55	8.08	7.97	0.84	C50
143	3.32	1.91	1.86	1.75	0.17	C53
163	3.79	2.18	1.60	1.58	0.20	C54-55
324	7.53	4.33	3.37	3.37	0.42	C56
—	—	—	—	—	—	C61
—	—	—	—	—	—	C62
229	5.32	3.06	1.46	1.47	0.13	C64-66, C68
137	3.19	1.83	0.87	0.88	0.07	C67
163	3.79	2.18	1.98	1.96	0.19	C70-C72
53	1.23	0.71	0.45	0.44	0.05	C73
302	7.02	4.04	2.68	2.59	0.29	C81-85, C88, C90, C96
229	5.32	3.06	2.14	2.08	0.22	C91-95, D45-47
380	8.83	5.08	3.17	3.16	0.33	Other
7 481	173.92	100.00	60.76	59.77	5.91	All
7 452	173.25	99.61	60.60	59.60	5.90	All sites exc. C44

附表5　2019年北京市郊区户籍居民恶性肿瘤发病主要指标

Appendix table 5　Incidence of all cancers in peri-urban areas of Beijing, 2019

部位 Site	男性 Male					
	例数 No. of cases	粗率 Crude rate （1/10⁵）	构成比 Freq. （%）	中标率 ASR China （1/10⁵）	世标率 ASR World （1/10⁵）	累积率 Cumulative rate （0~74，%）
口腔和咽Oral cavity & pharynx	163	6.14	1.62	3.29	3.25	0.40
鼻咽 Nasopharynx	19	0.72	0.19	0.50	0.48	0.04
食管 Esophagus	420	15.83	4.17	7.73	7.73	0.93
胃 Stomach	600	22.62	5.96	11.33	11.23	1.29
结直肠 Colon-rectum	1 409	53.12	13.99	27.00	27.03	3.23
肝 Liver	708	26.69	7.03	14.22	14.17	1.61
胆囊 Gallbladder	290	10.93	2.88	5.24	5.33	0.62
胰腺 Pancreas	257	9.69	2.55	4.85	4.85	0.58
喉 Larynx	126	4.75	1.25	2.38	2.46	0.30
肺 Lung	2 745	103.48	27.25	50.71	50.76	6.20
其他胸腔器官 Other thoracic organs	31	1.17	0.31	0.73	0.81	0.08
骨 Bone	44	1.66	0.44	1.30	1.18	0.10
皮肤恶性黑色素瘤 Cutaneous malignant melanoma	23	0.87	0.23	0.48	0.49	0.05
乳腺 Breast	10	0.38	0.10	0.18	0.19	0.02
子宫颈 Cervix	—	—	—	—	—	—
子宫体 Uterus	—	—	—	—	—	—
卵巢 Ovary	—	—	—	—	—	—
前列腺 Prostate	461	17.38	4.58	8.20	8.04	0.98
睾丸 Testis	15	0.57	0.15	0.54	0.56	0.04
肾及泌尿系统部位不明 Kidney & unspecified urinary organs	487	18.36	4.83	10.48	10.50	1.23
膀胱 Bladder	503	18.96	4.99	9.36	9.37	1.17
脑 Brain	157	5.92	1.56	4.23	4.24	0.40
甲状腺 Thyroid	608	22.92	6.04	21.46	17.43	1.49
淋巴瘤 Lymphoma	303	11.42	3.01	6.29	6.13	0.70
白血病 Leukemia	268	10.10	2.66	6.87	7.22	0.67
其他 Other	426	16.06	4.23	9.08	9.03	0.97
所有部位合计 All sites	10 073	379.73	100.00	206.47	202.48	23.13
所有部位除外皮肤 All sites exc. C44	9 962	375.54	98.90	204.15	200.25	22.91

女性 Female						
例数 No. of deaths	粗率 Crude rate （1/10⁵）	构成比 Freq. （%）	中标率 ASR China （1/10⁵）	世标率 ASR World （1/10⁵）	累积率 Cumulative rate （0~74，%）	ICD10
75	2.81	0.74	1.68	1.55	0.17	C00-10, C12-14
9	0.34	0.09	0.18	0.17	0.02	C11
117	4.38	1.16	1.66	1.72	0.17	C15
227	8.50	2.25	4.14	3.96	0.44	C16
975	36.51	9.66	17.98	17.46	2.04	C18-21
257	9.62	2.55	4.31	4.37	0.48	C22
213	7.98	2.11	3.43	3.34	0.33	C23-24
225	8.43	2.23	3.74	3.73	0.41	C25
7	0.26	0.07	0.10	0.11	0.01	C32
1 919	71.86	19.02	34.50	33.98	3.93	C33-34
20	0.75	0.20	0.43	0.41	0.05	C37-38
25	0.94	0.25	0.56	0.57	0.05	C40-41
23	0.86	0.23	0.48	0.43	0.05	C43
1 851	69.32	18.34	45.33	41.89	4.51	C50
257	9.62	2.55	6.89	6.01	0.60	C53
546	20.45	5.41	12.29	11.88	1.34	C54-55
292	10.94	2.89	6.71	6.44	0.71	C56
—	—	—	—	—	—	C61
—	—	—	—	—	—	C62
264	9.89	2.62	5.11	4.95	0.58	C64-66, C68
128	4.79	1.27	2.16	2.10	0.25	C67
115	4.31	1.14	2.96	2.88	0.26	C70-C72
1 689	63.25	16.74	56.68	47.86	4.19	C73
238	8.91	2.36	5.02	4.71	0.50	C81-85, C88, C90, C96
216	8.09	2.14	5.29	5.64	0.52	C91-95, D45-47
404	15.13	4.00	7.91	7.83	0.82	Other
10 092	377.93	100.00	229.54	214.00	22.42	All
9 983	373.85	98.92	227.68	212.16	22.22	All sites exc. C44

附表 6 2019 年北京市郊区户籍居民恶性肿瘤死亡主要指标

Appendix table 6 Mortality of all cancers in peri-urban areas of Beijing, 2019

部位 Site	男性 Male					
	例数 No. of deaths	粗率 Crude rate （1/10⁵）	构成比 Freq. （%）	中标率 ASR China （1/10⁵）	世标率 ASR World （1/10⁵）	累积率 Cumulative rate （0~74，%）
口腔和咽 Oral cavity & pharynx	96	3.62	1.64	1.72	1.82	0.23
鼻咽 Nasopharynx	24	0.90	0.41	0.57	0.54	0.04
食管 Esophagus	366	13.80	6.27	6.60	6.58	0.77
胃 Stomach	433	16.32	7.42	7.79	7.72	0.87
结直肠 Colon-rectum	569	21.45	9.75	10.21	9.99	0.88
肝 Liver	584	22.02	10.01	11.35	11.28	1.31
胆囊 Gallbladder	221	8.33	3.79	3.92	3.96	0.47
胰腺 Pancreas	237	8.93	4.06	4.42	4.34	0.49
喉 Larynx	58	2.19	0.99	1.00	1.00	0.10
肺 Lung	2 024	76.30	34.68	36.06	35.84	4.05
其他胸腔器官 Other thoracic organs	23	0.87	0.39	0.58	0.60	0.06
骨 Bone	26	0.98	0.45	0.55	0.51	0.05
皮肤恶性黑色素瘤 Cutaneous malignant melanoma	10	0.38	0.17	0.16	0.18	0.02
乳腺 Breast	4	0.15	0.07	0.07	0.08	0.01
子宫颈 Cervix	—	—	—	—	—	—
子宫体 Uterus	—	—	—	—	—	—
卵巢 Ovary	—	—	—	—	—	—
前列腺 Prostate	177	6.67	3.03	2.81	2.89	0.21
睾丸 Testis	1	0.04	0.02	0.06	0.05	0.00
肾及泌尿系统部位不明 Kidney & unspecified urinary organs	123	4.64	2.11	2.20	2.27	0.23
膀胱 Bladder	185	6.97	3.17	2.96	2.99	0.24
脑 Brain	108	4.07	1.85	2.62	2.49	0.25
甲状腺 Thyroid	16	0.60	0.27	0.32	0.31	0.03
淋巴瘤 Lymphoma	187	7.05	3.20	3.65	3.62	0.44
白血病 Leukemia	182	6.86	3.12	3.89	3.80	0.42
其他 Other	182	6.86	3.12	3.45	3.61	0.34
所有部位合计 All sites	5 836	220.00	100.00	106.97	106.46	11.50
所有部位除外皮肤 All sites exc. C44	5 812	219.10	99.59	106.56	106.02	11.48

例数 No. of deaths	粗率 Crude rate (1/10^5)	构成比 Freq. (%)	中标率 ASR China (1/10^5)	世标率 ASR World (1/10^5)	累积率 Cumulative rate (0~74, %)	ICD10
28	1.05	0.76	0.46	0.44	0.05	C00-10, C12-14
6	0.22	0.16	0.08	0.09	0.01	C11
86	3.22	2.35	1.19	1.21	0.09	C15
179	6.70	4.88	3.17	3.00	0.28	C16
375	14.04	10.23	5.94	5.88	0.51	C18-21
217	8.13	5.92	3.40	3.37	0.38	C22
198	7.41	5.40	3.04	3.02	0.33	C23-24
194	7.27	5.29	3.09	3.05	0.32	C25
3	0.11	0.08	0.03	0.03	0.00	C32
1 021	38.24	27.85	16.02	15.73	1.54	C33-34
8	0.30	0.22	0.13	0.14	0.01	C37-38
12	0.45	0.33	0.34	0.34	0.03	C40-41
9	0.34	0.25	0.17	0.16	0.01	C43
303	11.35	8.27	6.02	5.79	0.66	C50
101	3.78	2.76	2.05	1.97	0.19	C53
76	2.85	2.07	1.40	1.36	0.17	C54-55
162	6.07	4.42	3.12	3.09	0.36	C56
—	—	—	—	—	—	C61
—	—	—	—	—	—	C62
82	3.07	2.24	1.26	1.24	0.10	C64-66, C68
50	1.87	1.36	0.74	0.74	0.08	C67
115	4.31	3.14	2.27	2.22	0.23	C70-C72
22	0.82	0.60	0.34	0.33	0.03	C73
129	4.83	3.52	2.06	2.11	0.23	C81-85, C88, C90, C96
129	4.83	3.52	2.68	2.57	0.25	C91-95, D45-47
161	6.03	4.39	2.86	2.82	0.25	Other
3 666	137.29	100.00	61.85	60.71	6.11	All
3 644	136.46	99.40	61.57	60.41	6.09	All sites exc. C44

女性 Female

致谢
Acknowledgement

《2022 北京肿瘤登记年报》编委会对各医疗机构相关工作人员在本年报出版过程中给予的大力协助，尤其是国家癌症中心 / 全国肿瘤登记中心、北京市卫生健康委员会疾病预防控制处和北京市卫生健康大数据与政策研究中心在数据报送和质控等方面所做出的贡献，表示衷心感谢。

The editorial committee of *Beijing Cancer Registry Annual Report 2022* would like to express their gratitude to all staffs of medical institutions who have made a great contribution for the report, especially National Cancer Center & National Central Cancer Registry, Division of Disease Prevention and Control, Beijing Municipal Health Big Data and Policy Research Center, for their contribution on data reporting and quality control.